Pierre Mukadi Kaningu

Laboratory technicians and medical biologists

Pierre Mukadi Kaningu

Laboratory technicians and medical biologists

of the Democratic Republic of Congo, from the 1970s to the present day

ScienciaScripts

Imprint

Cover image: www.ingimage.com

This book is a translation from the original published under ISBN 978-620-6-71738-6.

Publisher:
Sciencia Scripts
is a trademark of
Dodo Books Indian Ocean Ltd. and OmniScriptum S.R.L publishing group

120 High Road, East Finchley, London, N2 9ED, United Kingdom
Str. Armeneasca 28/1, office 1, Chisinau MD-2012, Republic of Moldova, Europe
Printed at: see last page
ISBN: 978-620-7-90191-3

Table of contents

Acknowledgements

This dissertation was made possible with the support of the Conseil National des Biologistes Médicaux de la République Démocratique du Congo (CNBM-RDC).

I would like to thank once again the patriarchs of the CNBM, without whom much of this work would never have been written. I am referring in particular to the people in charge of the corporation from 1978 to the present day. Among these pioneers of the CNBM, I would mention Batangilayi (1er president of the Association de Techniciens de Laboratoire Médical du Zaïre (ATELAMEZ) and his collaborators Kabengele wa Kabenge, Mushiya wa Kalonji, Bitumba, Professor Kandolo Kakongo (honorary president of the CNBM), Muhoya (Honorary President of the CNBM), Fefe Baleka (Honorary President of the CNBM/ Kinshasa), Bembo Papy, Professors Lufuluabo Jean and Iyombe Jean-Paul and Malaba If Cléophas (Honorary Director of the Health Laboratories Department).

My thanks also go to all the medical biologists and laboratory technicians in the DRC who, from near and far, encouraged me to write down, for the first time, the life of the profession, including its history.

I cannot fail to acknowledge the efforts of President Bokabela for his encouragement and support throughout the dissertation process.

I would also like to express my gratitude to Kitenge Mateso, Mbuse Ilabo, Pukuta Nsimbu and Ngandu Muepu for their guidance during my short time in the laboratories of the Institut National de Recherche Biomédicale (INRB).

Finally, my thanks go to a lady, Dr Gaëlle OLLIVIER GOUAGNA, for her tireless efforts to support the laboratory system in the Democratic Republic of Congo, her availability and her support for the printing of this book.

It's difficult in these few lines to thank all the people who have encouraged me in this adventure. What can I say to them! Otherwise, I would like to express my sincere thanks and deep gratitude to all those who, from near or far, have contributed to the writing of this document.

Foreword

The profession of Laboratory Technician or Medical Biologist, which was once little-known and, above all, underestimated, is now taking on increasing importance with the surveillance of diseases, supported technically and financially by the World Health Organisation, among others, and the reinforced action in the field by the Centre for Disease Control (CDC) in Atlanta/United States of America.

A young biologist describes the history of this profession and the creation of higher education and university training, as well as the genesis and current development of the corporation that governs this profession, in a book entitled "*Techniciens de laboratoire et Biologistes Médicaux en République Démocratique du Congo, des années 1970 à nos jours*" (*Laboratory technicians and medical biologists in the Democratic Republic of Congo, from the 1970s to the present day)*.

This young Medical Biologist is called MUKADI KANINGU Pierre, who has had an exceptional career: first as a Laboratory Technician in 1999, then as a Medical Biologist in 2008 during his career at the Institut National de Recherche Biomédicale, and finally as a Doctor in Biomedical Sciences at the University of Lubumbashi. This is a model that should encourage other laboratory technicians and medical biologists to follow suit. Pursue university training in the era of the "Licence-Master-Doctorat" system in the Democratic Republic of Congo, or, as a health professional, write other documents that address other aspects while highlighting the profession, because, as the saying goes: "There is no such thing as a foolish profession, but there are only foolish people".

Dr. Denis KANDOLO KAKONGO

Medical Biologist (Microbiologist) Ordinary Professor

Introduction

The medical biology laboratory (MBL) is one of the areas of medical and health activity that plays the most important role, particularly in preventive, diagnostic, prognostic and therapeutic work. Generally located in a medical facility (health centre, hospital, clinic, etc.) or operating as an autonomous structure, the LBM draws on a wide range of skills, from the surface technician and other administrative staff to its main player, namely the laboratory technician (TL), the medical biologist (BM), the medical biologist or the pharmacist-biologist. It is not uncommon to find a psychologist, a veterinary surgeon, a chemist, etc. among the additional skills that the LBM needs today.

All these skills work in collaboration with each other, but also with other health professionals such as nurses, doctors and pharmacists, to carry out analyses, the results of which are the main and essential information needed to facilitate medical decision-making in a preventive, diagnostic, prognostic and therapeutic approach.

Context

As mentioned above, medical care and public health initiatives require the support of several health professionals. Among all these contributions, that of the TL or BM, via its laboratory, is essential, particularly in tropical regions with limited resources, such as the Democratic Republic of Congo (DRC), where infectious and parasitic diseases are endemic (Linsuke 2020). The COVID-19 pandemic, between 2020 and 2023, demonstrated that the BML is the key element in the detection and control of emerging infectious diseases (Fleming *2021*).

The DRC is constantly experiencing epidemics caused by viral, bacterial and parasitic diseases, for which biological diagnosis is essential. The endemicity of malaria, tuberculosis and acquired human immunodeficiency syndrome (AIDS) in the DRC also requires adequate laboratory services for biological surveillance and monitoring of medical care.

Thus, the main animator of the LBM in the DRC, the TL and/or BM, better his profession, is the focus of this dissertation. While in the majority of developed countries, the LBM is making great progress and the TL or BM enjoys satisfactory professional status, in many countries with limited resources such as the DRC, the LBM's regulations are aspirational, the professional association is struggling to establish its reputation, so that the prestige of belonging to this professional category is low.

In addition, there is confusion about names, the division of responsibilities and the qualifications/skills required. Very often, the LBM is marginalised and TLs/BMs live in constant frustration; they have the impression of being abandoned to their sad fate despite the increasingly relevant services they offer the community on a daily basis. As a result, the profession attracts few applicants, and the proportion of TL/BMs remains low in relation to national demand[1] .

Relevance

This document makes a modest contribution to all these concerns. In addition to information on the origins of TL and BM in the DRC, the evolution and development of the profession over the years, from 1976 to the present day, and all aspects of its environment in the DRC. Particular attention will be paid to the prospects for TL/BM. The main aim will be to describe the future LBM leader, taking account of current basic training in the DRC, which now applies the "Licence- Master- Doctorat" (LMD) system. But it will also be a question of arousing in young people the desire and ambition to serve the community as a TL or BM and to develop their profession as far as possible.

[1] There are currently around 9,378 TLs and BMs in the DRC, i.e. one TL/ BM for every 10,000 inhabitants (CNBM, 2023).

1 What we know about technical laboratory staff

Laboratory technical staff are divided into several categories according to their level of training, duties and responsibilities. For obvious reasons of mutual understanding and the needs of this book, the terms and definitions below will be considered.

Definitions of terms, vocabulary and concepts such as :

A laboratory technician, also known as a *"biomedical analysis technician"*, *"laboratory technologist"*, *"laboratory technologist"* or even *"laboratory technician"*, is a healthcare professional (member of the medical profession) responsible for carrying out medical analyses, including preparing the patient, taking samples, analysing and technically validating the results, in order to diagnose a disease.

At the end of their two- to three-year college or university training (Baccalaureate plus two or three years), depending on the country, they must have a sound knowledge of all branches of medical biology, including microbiology, cytology, haematology and clinical chemistry. He/she must demonstrate technical skills in the medical equipment used and in computer analysis tools. They must have certain qualities necessary for their work: for example, an excellent ability to analyse and summarise, enabling them to be relevant and precise when justifying the results they produce following the analyses carried out. They must also have a sound knowledge of hygiene, biosafety and biosecurity rules, so that they can apply them objectively, rigorously, methodically and organisationally.

In the DRC, the TL is available at levels A2 and A1.

- A2 level *laboratory technician*: qualified after four (4) years of secondary education in medical techniques (State Diploma level) and capable of correctly applying analytical techniques and procedures in the LBM.

- *A1* level *laboratory technician*: has three years' basic training at university level (Graduat) and, in addition to technical skills, is able to explain the whys and wherefores of things.

The medical biologist[2] is a healthcare professional specialising in medical analyses carried out on elements from the human body, most often biological fluids. They carry out and monitor medical biology procedures, and then interpret and validate the test results before they are released to the prescribing clinician and/or the patient, in order to contribute to medical diagnosis and patient follow-up in accordance with the rules of the Public Health Code. It is the link between the LBM and the parties involved (patients, clinicians and public health authorities).

To become a BM in the DRC, a two-year university course (Baccalaureate plus five years), consecutive to that of the TL (3 years), was required; but with the gradual implementation of the "*Licence- Master- Doctorat*" (LMD) system in 2021, the BM will be a TL who has completed a Master's degree in one of the branches of medical biology[3] . In addition to the skills of a TL, the BM must have mastery of the nomenclature of medical biology procedures, scientific and medical knowledge, the ability to interpret information, adapt to changes in technology and legislation, and team spirit.

In the DRC or elsewhere (Belgium, France, Canada, etc.), the "*medical biologist*" or "*pharmacist biologist*" becomes one after specialising for two to five years in one of the branches of medical biology.

Biotechnologist[4] ***(medical),*** "*Cell biologist*" or "*Molecular biologist*" is a healthcare professional who has mastered the diversity of structures, functions, reactions and behaviours of the living world. They must have the skills to develop (or modify) organisms such as cells, molecules or genes from plants or animals (plants, bacteria, viruses, parasites, insects, poultry, sheep, etc.) in order to meet

---

[2] https://www.studyrama.com/formations/fiches-metiers/sante/biologiste-medical-37484#formations
[3] ESU-RDC, 2022: Bachelor's and Master's degree models in healthsciences
[4] https://www.metiers-quebec.org/chimie/biotechno.html

specific needs for multiple applications (developing and perfecting vaccines, biological fertilisers, medical products, foods with improved nutritional qualities, etc.).

They may work in a research laboratory (biochemistry, microbiology or biotechnology), or in industry, supervising the staff and activities of a quality control department for manufactured products. He or she may also work in medical genetics as a specialist in the communication process focusing on the human problems associated with the onset or risk of onset of a genetic disease in a family and, in particular, the transmission of genetic information and support for individuals and families struggling with a hereditary disease.

Laboratory is an organisation with infrastructure, equipment, personnel and documentation for carrying out manipulations and experiments as part of scientific research, medical or materials analysis, technical testing or scientific and technical education.

The Association Congolaise des Laboratoires (ASCOLAB) sees the laboratory, in all fields, as the place par excellence for answering all the questions and concerns of a community.

A medical biology laboratory (MBL), *commonly referred to as a "clinical laboratory"* or *"medical laboratory"*, is designed to carry out biological, microbiological, immunological, biochemical, biophysical, cytological, immuno-haematological, haematological, anatomopathological, entomological, genetic or other examinations of substances of human origin in order to provide useful information for the diagnosis, management, prevention or treatment of diseases or the assessment of the state of health of human beings. The LBM can offer advice covering all aspects of laboratory examinations, including the interpretation of results and advice on other appropriate complementary examinations.

In accordance with the ministerial decree of 03 May 2003 on the organisation and operation of health laboratories in the DRC[5] , the mission of the LBMs is to :

- Providing diagnostic support for healthcare delivery services;
- Carrying out biomedical research to promote health ;
- Participate in quality control of services, goods and food;
- Facilitating training for healthcare professionals ;
- Contribute to epidemiological surveillance and
- Supporting research

And the new version of the ISO 15189 standard defines a laboratory as an entity responsible for the analysis of materials taken from the human body with the aim of providing information for diagnosis, monitoring, surveillance, prevention and treatment of disease, or assessment of health status.

As we said above, the TL and/or BM is the main competence in the organisation, operation and development of a LBM.

Conseil national des biologistes médicaux et techniciens de laboratoire de la République Démocratique du Congo (CNBM-RDC): Current name of the professional association of the main actors of the LBM (BM and TL) in DRC in accordance with the legal personality n°210/CAB/ME/MIN/J&GS/2022.

---

[5] Ministry of Health. Ministerial decree n°1250/ CAB/MIN/S/CJ/13/2003 of 03/05/2003 on the organisation and operation of health laboratories in the DRC.

2 The profession of laboratory technician and medical biologist in the Democratic Republic of Congo

2.1 *Overview*

In the early days of the profession, during the 1970s, and even today in some health areas of the country, medical biology is practised by people trained on the bench, nurses and medical staff other than TLs and BMs. Despite a significant increase in the number of TLs and BMs over the decades; from 34 TLs (first class in 1976) to some nine thousand three hundred and seventy-eight (9,378) currently listed by the CNBM[6] , this number remains insufficient for a country with an estimated population of around 100 million[7] .

As for the distribution according to level of education, the laboratory system in the DRC records around 85%, 15% and 0.4% who are respectively graduates, licentiates and holders of a master's degree or PhD (n = 9,378)[7] .

Due to inadequate organisation, it is difficult to obtain an estimate of the number of qualified TLs and BMs in the DRC. However, despite this, the DRC is far from meeting international requirements, which recommend one or two TLs per 10,000 inhabitants. Recent scientific surveys in Haut-Katanga and Equateur reported that 70.8% (n=479) and 70.9% (n=443) of laboratory providers respectively had not been trained at university[8] .

Furthermore, the working conditions of the TL and BM remain inadequate and do not allow the country's LBM system to perform effectively. The LBM is still the poor relation; you only have to travel around the country to see this (Fig.1). The reports of the few recent assessments show a relatively dilapidated and inadequate infrastructure, old and to some extent inappropriate equipment, major shortcomings in terms of staffing, quality assurance and biosafety (virtually non-existent analytical procedures), and the supply of reagents, culture media and other consumables. For

[6] Total number of full members of the CNBM (CNBM Directory, 2023).
[7] The last census in the DRC dates from 1984 (30 million inhabitants). In 2022, extrapolation gives 99,254,067 (https://countrymeters.info/fr/Democratic_Republic_of_the_Congo)
[8] Source: International centre for AIDS care and treatment program (ICAP)

example, of the 3,000 or so laboratories listed in the megalopolis of Kinshasa[9], only around 30 of them carry out bacterial cultures[10]. As far as staff are concerned, there is a lack of motivation, which is continually fuelled by underpayment and inadequate working conditions, including poor access to training and retraining.

Finally, as reported by LUFULUABO et *al*, *"the LBM resembles a diamond sorting plant where all the operators (cashiers, treasurers and others) are relatively satisfied, except for the miners who are the main producers of the precious stones"*. Meanwhile, thanks to their activities, TLs and BMs provide up to 80% of the figures throughout the medical process, but often receive modest bonuses that are disproportionate to their performance. The recent COVID-19 pandemic demonstrated the importance of the BML, which had been ignored for decades.

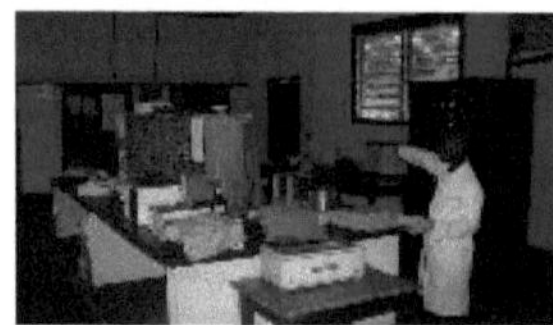
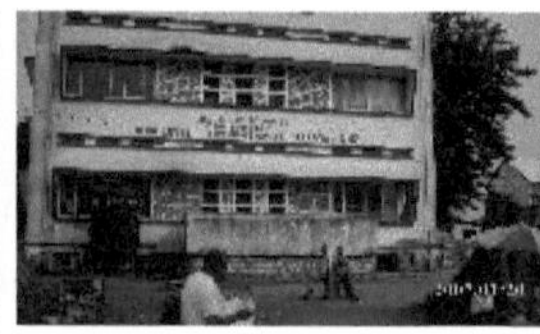
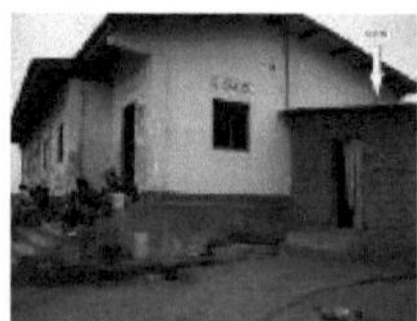

Figure 1: Medical laboratory (from left to right: HGR Bwamanda - Kananga Provincial Public Health Laboratory - CS de Boma Bungu)

Despite this gloomy picture of the profession, **a number of opportunities and individual experiences augur a bright future for TLs and BMs in the DRC.** We attempt to report them here:

- ***Increasing funding for the development of the BML*** in the context of epidemiological surveillance, operational research and also clinical research: certain epidemics such as Ebola and COVID-19, although causing sometimes irreversible damage, have nevertheless been opportunities for the development of the BML sub-sector. Support for biological diagnostics from the government and its partners during epidemics is often an opportunity to invest in and improve the laboratory system by building/rehabilitating infrastructure, renewing and modernising equipment, training service providers, and so on. To date, BMLs

[9] Source: Kinshasa Provincial Division

[10] Source: Bacteriology Department, French National Institute for Biomedical Research

located in the provinces are also capable of carrying out molecular biology analyses in real time (as in the provinces of Haut-Katanga, North Kivu, Lualaba and Ituri). As a result, some colleagues have seen their wallets swell considerably.

- Professional ***development***

While the majority of TLs and BMs work on the bench carrying out analyses, including those that were once very rare such as molecular biology, some TLs and BMs have secured professional development during and after which some are now qualified experts and researchers (with Master's and Doctorate degrees) in research institutes, universities and other regional and global organisations. Their areas of expertise include microbiology, field epidemiology, public health, quality management systems, biosafety and criminology.

Since the creation of the ISTM- Kinshasa, the TL and BM students trained there who continued on to the doctoral thesis have done so via other faculties other than that of Medicine in the DRC and other foreign university institutions. These include Professors Denis KANDOLO, Jean LUFULUABO, Nana MULENVO, Joseph MBASANI, Justine MBELU, Jacques MUZIAZIA, Thierry PALUKU, Jean-Paul IYOMBE, Jacquin KAMBALE and Jean-Pierre BASILUA.

But for the first time, it was at the Faculty of Medicine at the University of Lubumbashi, in July 2017 that BM Pierre MUKADI, trained at ISTM-Kinshasa, presented his doctoral thesis in the "Morpho-functional" stream of the Department of Biomedical Sciences, Faculty of Medicine at the University of Lubumbashi. Since then, a number of BMs have defended their theses at this Alma Mater. These include BM Philomène LUNGU, BM Erick KASAMBA and BM Kumel KUMELUNDU. The doctoral school at the ISTM in Kinshasa has also recently started training PhDs, particularly BMs.

- ***Business opportunities in the supply of*** equipment, materials, reagents, culture media and MBL inputs, in the ***creation of specialised private laboratories*** and in other types of services such as training, quality audit, coaching, etc. The following are just a few examples:

- The "***Surveillance Médicale***" and "**Emmaüs**" medical products sales companies, run by medical biologists Richard NGWANGU (Kinshasa-Gombe) and Bernard (Kisangani-Tshopo) respectively;
- Clément Ngonde's ***criminology laboratory*** in Kinshasa-Gombe;
- SARLU "***Cabinet MK***", for the design and installation of laboratories, technical training, accreditation support, auditing, etc. in Kinshasa and Lubumbashi, by BM Pierre MUKADI.

2.2 *History of the profession*

The genesis of the TL and BM professions in the DRC is totally dependent on ISTM-Kinshasa.

The ISTM-Kinshasa was the first institution of higher medical education, created in May 1973. As we shall see below, it should be noted that before the ISTM was founded, several medical colleges in Kinshasa offered courses in the medical-social field, but did not yet train TLs.

The threefold mission of the current ISTM-Kinshasa can be summed up as follows[11] :

- Train managers specialising in medical and paramedical sciences and techniques;
- To organise research into the adaptation of new techniques and technologies to the conditions of the DRC and to confer legal degrees in accordance with the legal and regulatory provisions on the award of academic degrees;
- Giving back to the community.

In addition, two other medical teaching institutions, at secondary level, were created: (1) the Institut de Technique Médicale de Tshikaji (ITM), whose origins lie in the Institut Médical Chrétien du Kasaï founded in 1954 in Lubondai and which moved later in the 1970s to Tshikaji, 15 kilometres south of Kananga in what is now the province of Kasaï, and (2) the Institut Médical

[11] Source: ISTM-Kinshasa, http://istmkin.education/fr/historique-istm-kinshasa/

Evangélique de Kimpese (IME) in the province of Kongo Central. These two institutions began to deliver A2 level TLs in 1978 (Fig.2). Among the main institutions at this level is the national pilot institute for the teaching of health sciences (INPESS) in Kinshasa (formerly the Kinshasa medical teaching institute - IEMK - a victim of the systematic looting of 1991-1993) which, after renovation in 2013, trains pharmacy assistants, midwives, nurses, sanitation technicians and medical and public health laboratory technicians.

TLs and BMs are currently trained in a number of public and private higher education and university institutions across the country.

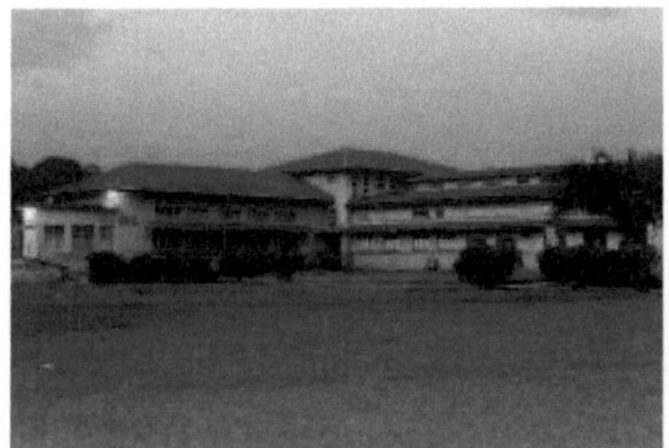

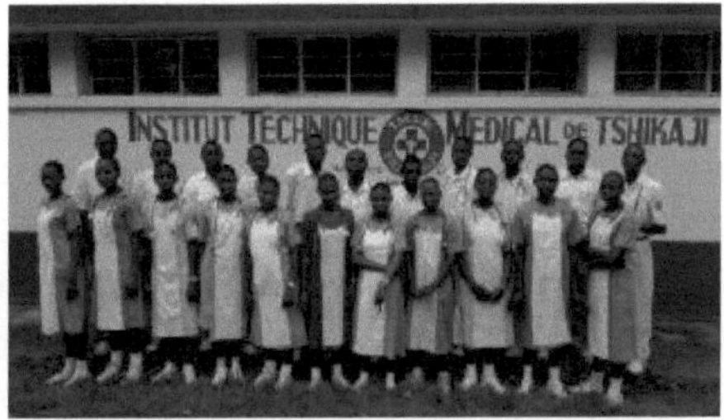

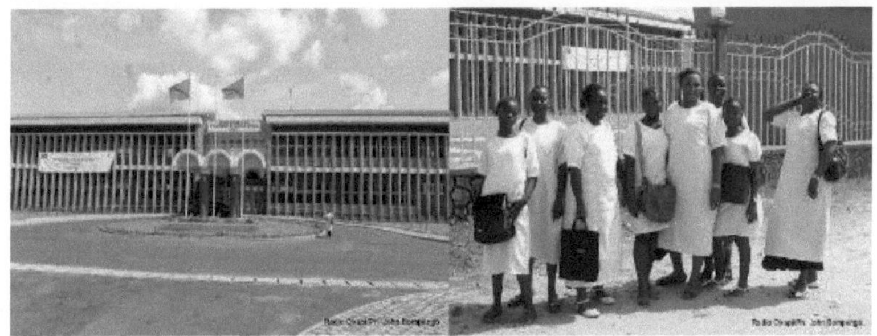

Figure 2: From left to right, Institut médical évangélique de Kimpese - Institut technique médical de Tshikaji and Institut national pilote d'enseignement des sciences de santé de Kinshasa.

2.2.1 *Genesis of the Institut Supérieur de Techniques Médicales*

In order to present the history of the profession, we interviewed in turn some of those whom we consider to be "Pioneers" and resource persons of the profession (Appendix 1). Following the individual interviews with each of these pioneers and pillars, we have compiled and summarised their testimonies as follows:

As early as 1973, a faculty institute, the Institut supérieur des études paramédicales (ISEPM), attached to the Faculty of Medicine of the Université Nationale du Zaïre (UNAZA), Kinshasa campus (now the University of Kinshasa), was organising courses in Hospital Management and Nursing Sciences. This institute was created by decision of the UNAZA Revolutionary Council, held in the city of Kisangani in May 1973. Dr Carlo ROSSETI (a former expert from the World Health Organisation, WHO) and the Belgian cooperation agency were responsible for lobbying for its creation. In 1974, the ISEPM became the "Institut Supérieur de Techniques médicales" (ISTM), by decision of the Political Bureau of the People's Revolutionary Movement (MPR). Dr Carlo ROSSETI and Maitre ABANGADGAPAKWA became the first Director General and Secretary General respectively. This is how the ISTM obtained its management autonomy and separated from the Faculty of Medicine at the UNAZA Kinshasa campus. Very quickly, during the same academic year 1973-1974, in response to the country's needs, the "Kinesitherapy", "Radiology" and "Laboratory Techniques" sections were created and around 150 students enrolled in all three sections combined.

However, as far as its infrastructure was concerned, the ISTM continued to operate in the buildings of the Faculties of Law and Agronomy on the campus of what is now the University of Kinshasa (UNIKIN). In the 2000s, ISTM began moving to its own campus on Route Kimwenza, opposite the psychiatric hospital known as the "Centre Neuro-psycho-pathologique de l'UNIKIN". Since then, buildings have gradually been erected to house the application laboratory, auditoriums, offices and, later in 2012, the general management, before leaving the UNIKIN campus for good. Today, ISTM-Kinshasa is a campus in continuous development, both in terms of buildings and equipment, particularly for the "Laboratory Techniques" section.

Similarly, due to a shortage of professors and other members of the teaching staff, the ISTM continues to use professors from the faculties of Medicine, Science and Pharmacy from other local and foreign university institutions. To date, the ISTM has sixty-four[12] professors, an increasing number of whom have been trained or are in the process of being trained thanks to the ISTM's partnership with national and international academic institutions.

2.2.2 *Background to the Laboratory Techniques course*

During the 1973-1974 academic year, the Laboratory Techniques section at ISTM Kinshasa enrolled several dozen students in the first year of their degree course. More than 60 of them went on to the second year, and only 34 out of 35 completed the 3-year course in 1976. Among them were some pioneers whom we interviewed in the course of writing this book.

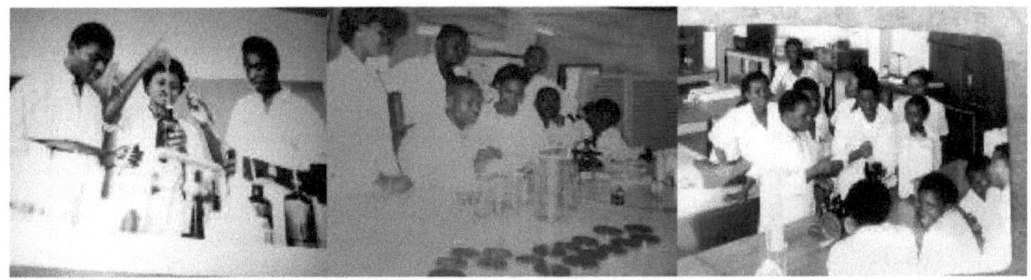

Figure 3: Archive images of practical work by chemistry and microbiology students at ISTM-Kinshasa

The TL training programme, inspired by the Canadian and Belgian programmes of the time, included common core courses with students from other sections, but also and above all specific and practical courses dedicated solely to future TLs. The ISTM-Kinshasa had teaching laboratories for the specific fields of Chemistry and Microbiology, as well as a microscopy room where each student had his or her own microscope for practical work.

The teachers were WHO experts and other teachers and professors from the UNAZA Faculty of Medicine, Kinshasa campus. We can mention in particular Dr Firmin KRUBWA (Microbiologist at the UNAZA Faculty of Medicine, Kinshasa campus, and who was the first head of the "Laboratory" section from 1973-1978), Mr KELLENS, second head of the Laboratory section between 1978 and 1982 (Table 1).

To complete their academic training, the first future TLs carried out their annual academic placements under the

[12] Source: ISTM-Kinshasa, December 2023

supervision of the laboratory assistants of the time (nurses and other service providers trained in the laboratory by Belgian experts towards the end of colonisation).

In the early days of basic TL training, a percentage > 55% was required to qualify for the next year. So, for example, Mr *Dangala*, Mr *Oledi* and Mr *Baelongadi* were obliged to repeat the 2ème year of graduation to find themselves part of the 2ème class of TLs of 1977.

Table 1: Heads of the Laboratory Techniques section, ISTM-Kinshasa

N°	Names	Period	Photo
1	Prof. Firmin KRUBWA	1973 - 1978	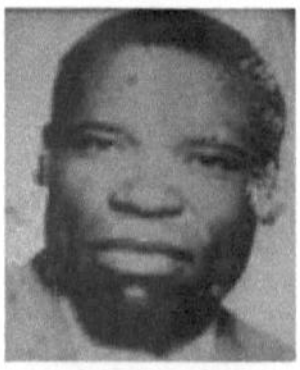
2	Prof. KELLENS	1978 - 1982	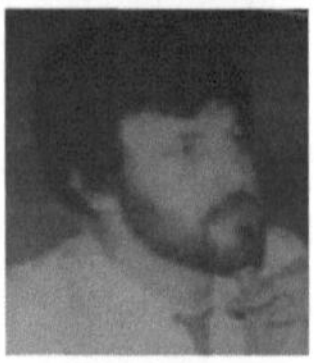
3	C.T. HERABO MANGILIO	1982- 1986 1994 - 1995	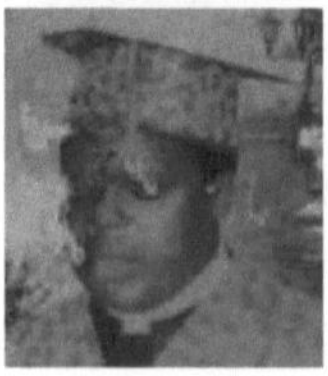

4	Prof. KANDOLO KAKONGO	1986 - 1994	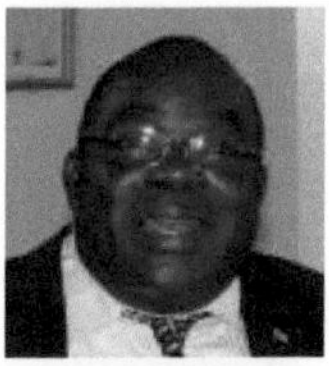
5	Prof. MPONA MINGA MISHIMA	1995 - 1997	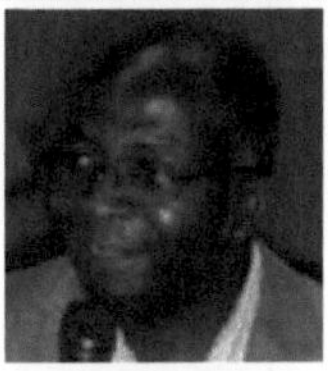
6	C.T. KANDOLO MUGALU	1997 - 2000	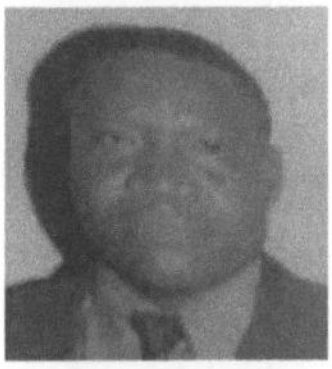
7	Prof. NKEBOLO MALAFU	2000 - 2006	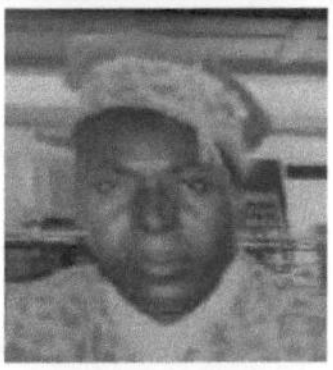
8	Prof. NDONGA LUTUMBA	2006 - 2010	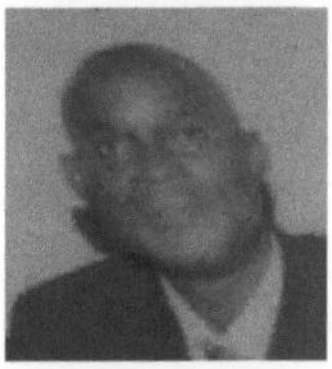
9	C.T. MBADU ZEBE	February - October 2010	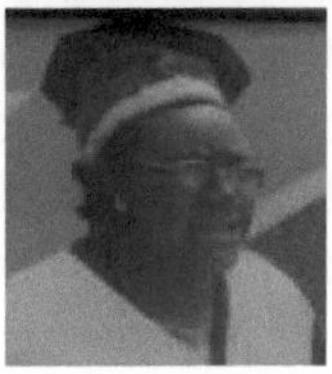

10	C.T. NTAKOYI NKOMU	2010 -2016	
11	Prof. BASILUA KANZA	2016 - 2021	
12	Prof. IYOMBE ENGEMBE	2021 - 2023	
13	Prof. MBASANI MANSI	2023 -	

At the end of these first three years of basic training in laboratory techniques, only 34 successful candidates passed their end-of-cycle exams and qualified as TLs. All the successful candidates were requisitioned and employed in higher and university education (Kinshasa University Clinics, the UNAZA Faculty of Medicine and the ISTM), in health institutions such as the current Centre Hospitalier Universitaire Renaissance - Ex. Maman Yemo - in Kinshasa, the Clinique Kinoise, the Bakwanga Mining Health Service and in the national army. Most of these first TLs were recruited even before completing their final year at the ISTM, because they were the very first and the community was waiting impatiently for them. However, some were retained as "Chargés des Pratiques Professionnelles" with a view to continuing their training right up to the doctoral thesis; these included the current Professor Dénis KANDOLO KAKONGO and the Chef des Travaux (CT) Marcel KABENGELE WA KABENGE. Other TLs were recommended to the Institut Louis Pasteur in Paris, France, for specialisation, including Elisabeth MUSHIYA WA KALONJI, KALUME, KIAMBEZI and FALANKA. This specialisation was a prelude to the training of senior technicians to work in the laboratories of the National Institute for Biomedical Research (INRB), which was in the process of being set up.

2.3 *Start of the second cycle of medical biology*

The first graduating class in Laboratory Techniques completed its three-year course in 1976. A total of 56 of the very first TLs trained in the DRC were poured into the job market, which was still untapped at the time. At the time, the ISTM-Kinshasa had planned to organise the second cycle, i.e. the Bachelor's degree in Medical Biology, two years later, starting in the 1978-1979 academic year; but this did not happen for a number of obvious reasons that we will attempt to explain in the following paragraphs.

It was only in 1998 that the ISTM-Kinshasa obtained the necessary authorisation to finally organise Bachelor's degree courses in Medical Biology (Fig.4). Only a small group of the country's very first TLs returned to the ISTM to realise the dream of the 'Licence'. But what happened during all those long years of impatience? Why didn't the ISTM obtain this authorisation until twenty-two years later?

It is well known that in the country of Patrice Emery Lumumba, politics has infiltrated every area of Congolese life since the years of the *Mobutian* dictatorship. Resistance from certain medical bodies at the time also delayed the advent of the Bachelor's degree in Medical Biology at ISTM-Kinshasa.

In addition, it was not until a number of events took place, in particular the lobbying carried out several years earlier by a group of members of the Association de Techniciens de Laboratoire Médical du Zaïre (ATELAMEZ), including Sieur Jean-François FEFE BALEKA, and the advent of Professor Dénis KANDOLO KAKONGO at the head of the ISTM-Kinshasa management committee between 1997 and 2000, that authorisation was finally obtained from the Minister responsible for higher and university education (ESU) to organise the second cycle at ISTM-Kinshasa, to finally obtain authorisation from the Minister for Higher and University Education (ESU) to organise the second cycle at ISTM Kinshasa. Despite opposition from certain medical bodies right up to the last minute, the degree course opened its doors, initially not only in Medical Biology, but also in Nursing. Then, over the years, other sections implemented the Bachelor's degree.

It should be noted that, as with the training programme for graduates in laboratory techniques, the training programme for bachelor's degrees has been designed on the basis of programmes from other internationally renowned universities, such as those in Canada (Université de Québec) and Belgium (Louvain, Liège and Université libre de Bruxelles).

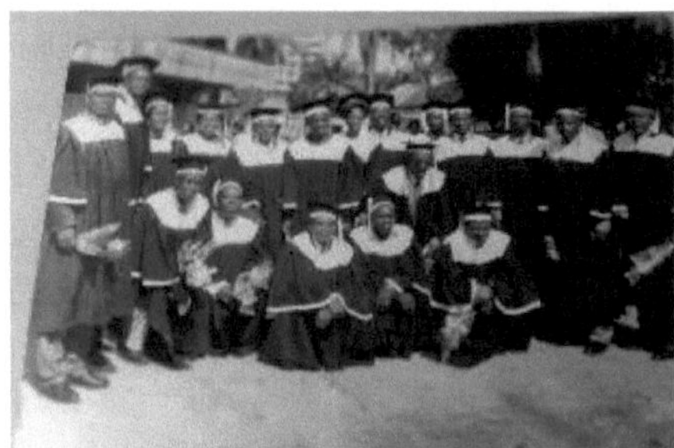

Figure 4: *First class of medical biology graduates, ISTM- Kinshasa, 2001*

All ten sections currently organised at ISTM-Kinshasa are: (1) Medical Biology, (2) Management of Health Organisations, (3) Hygiene, Occupational Health and Environmental Management, (4) Medical Imaging, (5) Midwifery, (6) Community Health, (7) Nursing, (8) Motor and Rehabilitation Sciences, (9) Food Science, Nutrition and Dietetics, and (10) Pharmaceutical Techniques.

In addition, the ISTM-Kinshasa Doctoral School, created in 2015, had started its activities concretely during the 2016-2017 academic year with a Master's programme for Medical Biology and Nursing Sciences. Then, in the second academic year 2017-2018, for Community Health (Biostatistics), Food Science, Nutrition and Dietetics, and Management of Health Organisations. It should be noted that the Masters in Medical Biology are currently organised for *Biochemistry-Clinical Chemistry*, *Haematology-Immunohaematology* and *Medical Microbiology*.

Now that it is capable of training its own PhDs, the ISTM-Kinshasa aims to become a university called the "*Haute école de sciences de la santé*".

2.4 *Overview of the trade association*

2.4.1 *Association of Laboratory Technicians of Zaire, ATELAMEZ (1978 - 1986)*

The professional association of laboratory technicians was quickly set up by the TLs of the first graduating class in Laboratory Techniques (July 1976). They quickly set up the Association of Laboratory Technicians of Zaire (ATELAMEZ) on 18 March 1978.

Here are the main events and opportunities that led to the creation of ATELAMEZ:

- ***Urgent need for laboratory technicians in companies and hospitals in Leopoldville (present-day Kinshasa) and throughout the country***
  As described in section 2.2.2 above, the first TLs, who were quickly recruited by the user institutions, were assimilated by default to nurses in terms of pay and other social benefits. As a result, frustrations began to manifest themselves, and the TLs very quickly sought to organise themselves into a trade union or professional organisation in order to better express and present their demands as a body different from doctors, nurses, in short other health professionals.
- ***Lack of laboratory experts at the World Health Organisation country office***
  In this context, the WHO, which had also campaigned for the creation of the ISTM, was suffering from a lack of local experts in its Kinshasa office, as well as a health laboratory contact.

This is how the idea of creating an association began to cross the minds of the TLs. It all began with meetings of a trade union nature to deal with the frustration of TLs in hospitals. Encouraged in particular by the WHO and their former trainers at the ISTM, the group of ATELAMEZ pioneers succeeded in organising the corporation's very first event with the support of the WHO and the Ministry of Health. A seminar was organised in 1978, bringing together TLs, delegates from the WHO, the Ministries of Health and Higher and University Education. This event helped to raise awareness and consolidate the nascent association.

The movement was thus strengthened and the very first national committee of the corporation was set up, by consensus, in 1978. The members of this committee included the very first national president, Aloïs BATANGILAYI MESU, and the secretaries Marcel KABENGELE WA KABENGE and Elisabeth MUSHIYA WA KALONJI.

From then on, the organisation of ATELAMEZ continued with sporadic meetings and activities, the main ones being :

- The ***first seminar***, mentioned above, introduced ATELAMEZ to the Ministry of Health and the WHO;
- The fight for ***adequate fees for TLs*** and other non-medical health professionals. At the time, faced with the President of the Medical Association, President Batangilayi was able to fight for the payment of adequate fees, in addition to the Congolese state salary, to members of all the non-physician guilds. All the other public sector hospitals gradually implemented this system of payment of fees, also for non-medical health professionals. It should be noted that even in the early days of the profession, TLs pointed out that they did most of the work in the medical care process.
- ***Recognition as an entity in its own right***: this took place during a meeting organised by Professor KALENGAYI (Faculty of Medicine, Kinshasa campus/ UNAZA) in the conference room of the Ministry of Foreign Affairs in Kinshasa.

ATELAMEZ also played a part in the creation of INRB. Some ATELAMEZ members, including BM Elisabeth MUSHIYA WA KALONJI, were selected for further training at the Institut Louis Pasteur in Paris, France, as they needed senior technicians to work in the future public health laboratory, INRB.

After a few years of management, in 1986 the BATANGILAYI committee organised a meeting at the ISTM, the legendary headquarters of ATELAMEZ, at the end of which Professor Dénis KANDOLO was appointed President of ATELAMEZ by consensus.

2.4.2 *Conseil national des Techniciens de Laboratoire, CNTL (1991-2001)*

As soon as he took up his post in 1986, Professor Dénis KANDOLO, thanks to his reputation, his position at the WHO, his creative spirit and his address book, began to raise awareness among TLs throughout the country and succeeded in setting up provincial committees, particularly in Shaba (the former province of Katanga) and in Kinshasa, where Darius SELEMANI UNGU of happy memory and Jean-François FEFE BALEKA were the first provincial presidents. At the time, many TLs were not interested in the corporation and in most cases, some committee members were either "single candidates" or cronies.

In 1990, an elective assembly was held at national level and Professor Dénis KANDOLO, the sole candidate, was elected President of the CNTL National Committee. BAELONGANDI BOLIO and MUHOYA DJUNGAYANE became Vice-Chairman and Secretary General respectively. The two main objectives of this committee were (i) to obtain legal status and (ii) to create a Bachelor's degree in laboratory techniques at ISTM-Kinshasa.

The committee had the merit of being officially installed at a major ceremony held in the Palais du peuple conference room, attended by members of the CNTL, several political and academic authorities, delegations of partners from the Ministry of Health and other local dignitaries. Société commerciale et industrielle Bemba du Zaïre (SCIBE-Zaïre) was the main sponsor of this historic ceremony.

The CNTL also formally participated in the Sovereign National Conference[13] . Sieur ONALUNDULA of happy memory, an

[13] The Sovereign National Conference (August 1991 to December 1992) marked the start of a long period of political transition in Zaire. It brought together 2,800 representatives of 200 political parties and professional associations from all over the country.

INRB agent at the time, was one of the 2,800 participants in one of the greatest events in the post-colonial history of the Belgian Congo in 1991.

During this same period (1991-1992), a fortnightly newsletter was published thanks to the creative spirit of Works Manager François DANGALA.

The main allies of president Dénis KANDOLO were BM Papy MUHOYA and Jean-François FEFE, vice-president of the national committee and provincial president of the city of Kinshasa respectively. It was thanks to this team that the CNBM's first articles of association were drawn up in 2001, and the F92 was obtained[14] later.

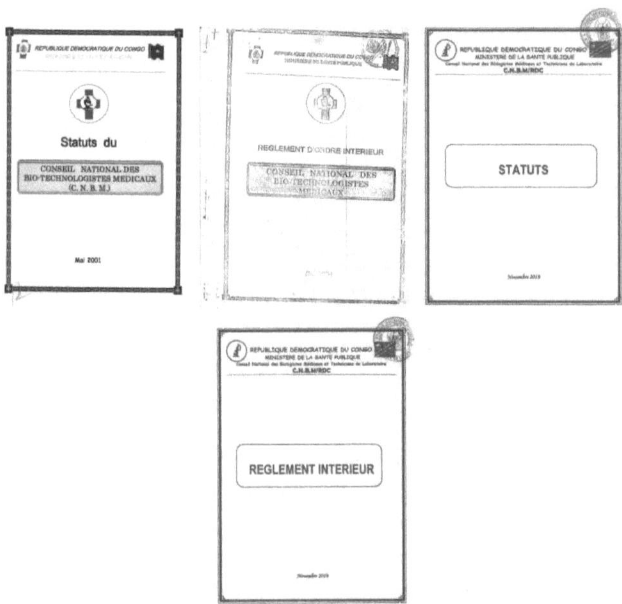

Figure 5: *Successive statutes of the CNBM between 2001 and 2020*

[14] F92: Provisional authorisation to operate a non-profit association granted by the Ministry of Justice

2.4.3 *National Council of Medical Biotechnologists, CNBM (2001-2018)*

MUHOYA DJUNGAYANE" Committee, 2001 - 2014

Shortly after the year 2000, the activities of the corporation began to sink into lethargy, notably due to the unavailability of the national professor-president, who was now posted outside the country by his main employer, the WHO. So it was that in 2001, an awakening of the still-active members led to the organisation of a major General Assembly (GA) at the ISTM-Kinshasa (the legendary headquarters of the corporation since its creation). At the end of this AGM, BM Papy MUHOYA was appointed, by consensus, interim president of the national committee in order to revitalise activities and develop the corporation. The "MUHOYA" committee relied heavily on the Kinshasa provincial committee to organise the CNBM, in particular by setting up CNBM units in the capital's main medical facilities and also by actively collecting subscriptions from full members.

During this period, a number of medical facilities in the city of Kinshasa stood out for their dedication to the CNBM; these were mainly the Cliniques Ngaliema, the INRB, the Cliniques universitaires de Kinshasa and the ISTM-Kinshasa.

During this period, the CNBM's national headquarters were moved to the *Matonge* district in the commune of *Kalamu*, and monthly meetings of the provincial committee were held. One of the main results of this committee was the formal recognition of the CNBM as the "Conseil National des Biotechnologistes Médicaux" by the Ministry of Health, as well as obtaining document "F 92" from the Ministry of Justice, authorising the corporation to operate officially, pending legal personality.

It was also during this period that the first membership card, signed by Professor KANDOLO, then President, was issued to all full members of the CNBM, including those from the provinces (Fig.6).

After these few attempts to revitalise the CNBM, there was finally a second period of inactivity, which lasted until just before 2009.

Concerned by the situation, a movement of colleagues took it upon themselves to help change things by organising themselves into a think tank to revitalise the CNBM's activities, led by TL Papy BEMBO. Buoyed by this pressure, Professor-President Denis KANDOLO convened a general meeting in September 2009, at the end of which a new provisional national committee was formed by consensus, with the task of reorganising the association and organising general elections; BM Kadhafi SUMBA was its chairman.

However, the ad-interim committee supported by the Kinshasa provincial committee will not accept these resolutions, hence the duality at the top of the CNBM.

A group of wise men was called in to reconcile the two groups. A harmonisation meeting chaired by the Director of Laboratories at the time, BM If Cléophas MALABA, led to harmonisation by merging the two committees: Papy MUHOYA and Kadhafi SUMBA.

Putting the interests of the profession above all else, the members of the harmonised committee have carried out a titanic task that will culminate in 2014 in the organisation of elections leading to a democratic transfer of power between the outgoing MUHOYA committee and the incoming KANYONGA committee.

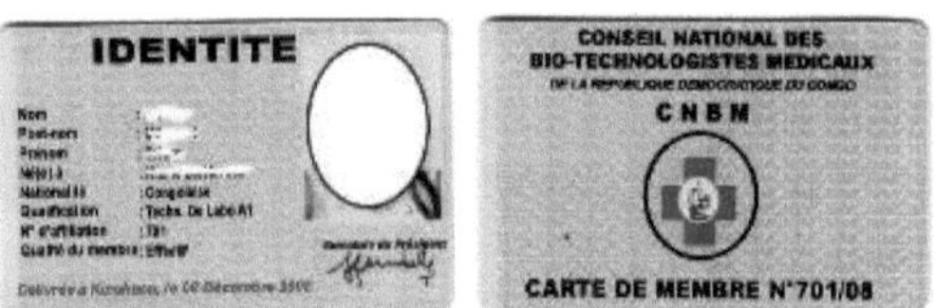

Figure 6: *CNBM membership card between 2001 and 2015*

KANYONGA MANUELE" Committee, 2014- 2018

In 2012, there was a new awakening, and this time many successive meetings were held at the Bondeko clinic, thanks to BM Papy EKOFEMBE. An electoral commission was set up under the chairmanship of BM Antoine MANGAMBA. Preparations for the elections continued until the beginning of 2014.

Two thousand and fourteen marks the start of a new era within the CNBM. The first elections for members of the CNBM national committee, extended to the provinces, were held on 16/03/2014 in the large, packed meeting room at the *Lindonge* centre in Limete, Kinshasa. These elections had the merit of also including the country's provinces, via the CNMB's provincial officers. The late Professor Pascal KANYONGA MANUELE's committee was elected, with BM Pierre MUKADI and Papy BEMBO as vice-presidents for a 4-year term.

The KANYONGA committee has left its mark on the history of the CNBM, notably through the acquisition of the CNBM's first national headquarters, which was fully equipped and employed a secretariat working 6 to 8 hours a day. This first official headquarters of the CNBM was located on the historic avenue de l'Université n°203/6, in the commune of Lemba in Kinshasa, between January 2015 and June 2018. The design and colour of the CNBM's membership card were also improved during the same period (Fig.7).

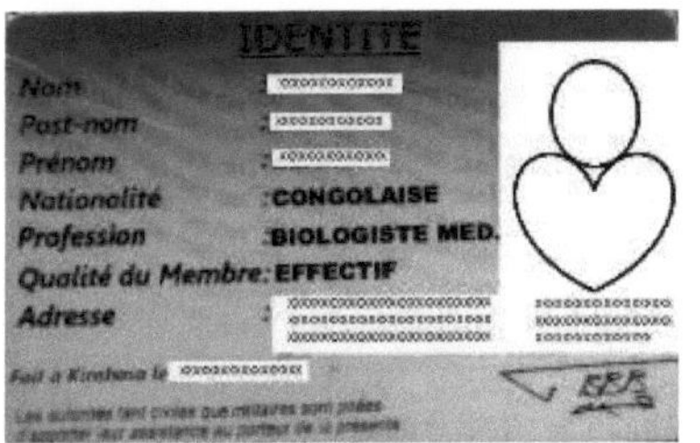

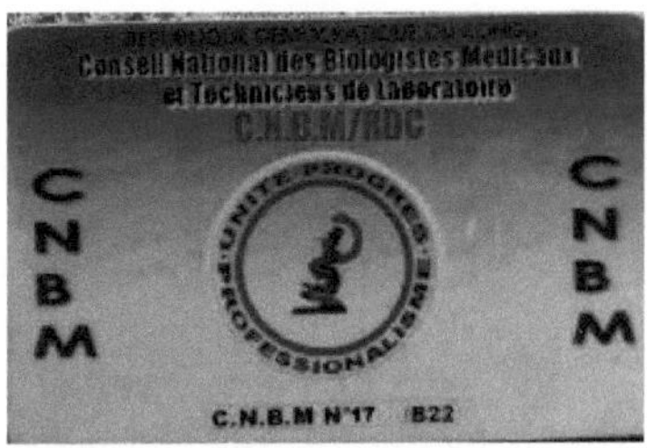

Figure 7: *CNBM full membership card between 2015 and 2019*

The other merit of the KANYONGA MANUELE committee was the respect of its 4-year mandate as stipulated by the CNBM statutes. Indeed, this committee organised the elections during the elective Assembly of 28 October 2018, at the end of which new members were elected, including BM BOKABELA BALAMBA as national president.

2.4.4 *National Council of Medical Biologists and Laboratory Technicians, CNBM (2018-)*

BOKABELA BALAMBA" Committee, 2018-

At the end of the mandate of the national committee chaired by Professor KANYONGA, elections were again held on 28 October 2018 in Kinshasa. Some provinces such as Central Kongo, Kwango, Kwilu, North Kivu, South Kivu, etc. sent their representatives. The elections were held in conjunction with the CNBM's second ethics days (Fig. 8).

République Démocratique du Congo
Conseil National des
Bio-technologistes Médicaux
"C.N.B.M"
Deuxièmes Journées
Déontologiques
Thème:
Validation
des résultats d'analyses biomédicales
Assemblée élective des membres
du bureau du Comité National

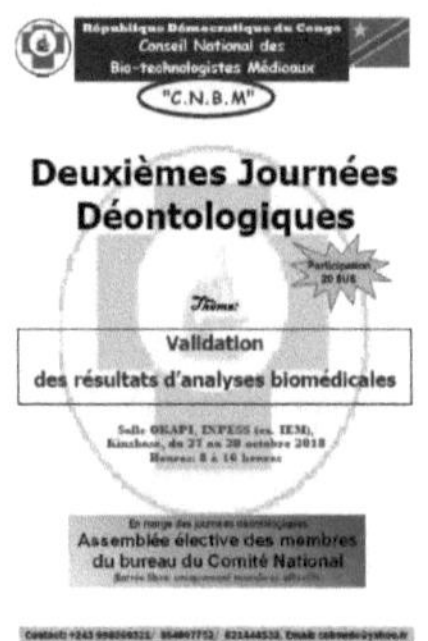

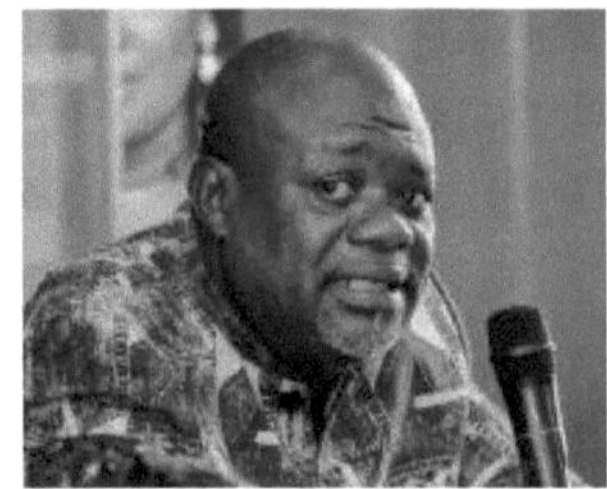

Figure 8: Poster for the second CNBM ethics days chaired by BM Blandin Bokabela, President of the CNBM (2018-)

Shortly after its installation, the new committee led by President BOKABELA completed the revision of the Articles of Association undertaken by the KANYONGA committee.

It should be noted that the revised name of the corporation is now the "Conseil National des Biologistes Médicaux et Techniciens de laboratoires", or CNBM for short. In 2019, the CNBM's revised statutes were notarised for the first time. And shortly before the end of their first mandate, the "BOKABELA" committee obtained the "Legal Personality" of the CNBM whose number: *Min. Justice n°210/CAB/ME/MIN/J&GS/2022*.

After the re-election of almost all the members of the "BOKABELA" committee in 2022, the bill creating the order of BMs and TLs has finally been validated and is currently being sent to parliament, via the National Assembly, for possible adoption during the September 2023 session (Fig.9).

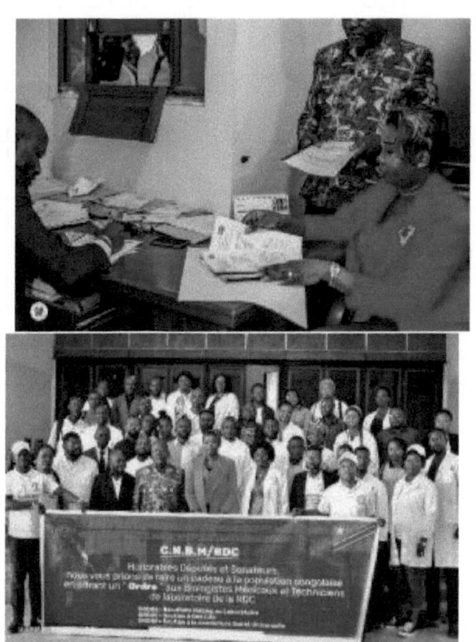

Figure 9: Filing of the bill to create the DRC's BM and TL order by MP Christelle Vuanga, Kinshasa, 9 June 2023

Table 2: Presidents of the TL and BM corporation in the Democratic Republic of Congo

N°	Names	Period	Photo
1	Aloïs BATANGILAYI MESU	1978 - 1986	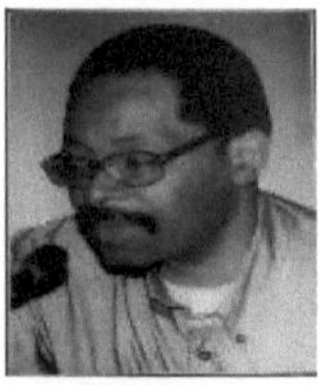
2	Dénis KANDOLO KAKONGO	1986 - 2001	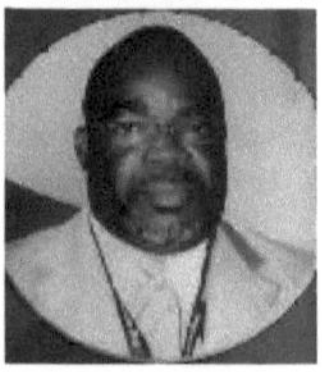
3	Papy MUHOYA DJUNGAYANE	2001 - 2014	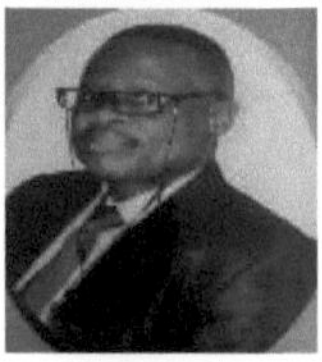
4	Pascal MANUELE KANYONGA	2014 - 2018	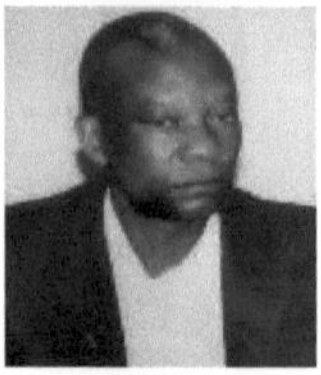
5	Blandin BOKABELA BALAMBA	2018 -	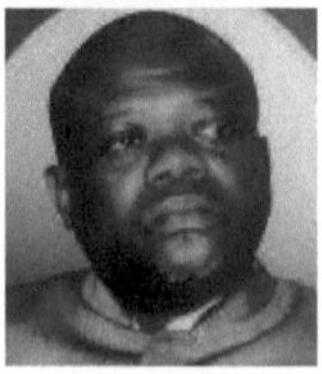

2.5 ***Stakeholders of the Medical Biology Laboratory in the Democratic Republic of Congo***

2.5.1 *Health Laboratories Division (DLS)*

In the DRC, the LBM is organised at the highest level via the Direction des Laboratoires de Santé (DLS), which currently operates within the General Secretariat of the Ministry of Public Health, Hygiene and Prevention. The DLS was known as the "8ème directorate" before the reforms introduced in 2017.

The origins of the DLS date back to the 1990s, when it was part of the former "Pharmacy, Medicines and Laboratory Directorate (3rd Directorate)", within which the fifth division was responsible for laboratories. A few years later, following an internal reform, this 5ème division included (i) the public health laboratory, (ii) the public health laboratory and (iii) blood transfusion. During the same period, a first attempt was made to create a Laboratory Department with 3 divisions: (i) Public Health Laboratory, (ii) Public Health Laboratory and (iii) Blood Transfusion. However, this attempt was unsuccessful and the three divisions were once again attached to the 3ème Directorate.

Shortly before 2003, Professor Dénis KANDOLO, with the support of the WHO and other stakeholders, worked to hold the first general health conference, at the end of which decree N°CAB/FP/JMK/PP/044/2003 of 28 March 2003, signed by the late Professor MASHAKO MAMBA, organised the BML sub-sector in the DRC for the first time.

Following the reform that took place that same year, the Organisational Framework of the Ministry of Health was modified with the creation of 13 Directorates, among which the DLS was henceforth counted as 8ème Directorate. As a reminder, the BM If Cléophas MALABA MUNYANJI , former Head of Division in the 3ème Directorate, was the very first Director of the 8ème Directorate.

The 2017 health sector reform restructured the health administration into directorates-general and the DLS was organised within the Direction Générale de Lutte contre la Maladie (DGLM). At the time, recruitment was organised in line with international standards, and BM If Cléophas MALABA MUNYANJI was once again selected as Director and Head of Services of the new DLS. In November 2022, after several decades at the head of the DLS, BM If Cléophas MALABA MUNYANJI was promoted to Secretary General for Communication and Media and one of his collaborators, the Head of Division, BM Justin KINZIANGU MAWINA, assumes this responsibility to this day.

Currently the DLS, which is the eye of the Ministry of Health, has as its main mission the management of all aspects of the LBM, including the organisation of the laboratory system in the DRC. In particular, it is responsible for policies, regulations and resource planning for (i) public health laboratories; (ii) clinical analysis laboratories; (iii) blood banks; (iv) medical product sales outlets (reagents, materials and medical equipment); and (v) quality control of drinking water and foodstuffs. To do this, it relies on the technical expertise of the INRB and the national laboratories of specialised programmes such as the National Tuberculosis Programme (PNLT) and the National HIV-AIDS Programme (PNLS), all of which form its "technical arm". The DLS currently comprises three divisions: (1) Clinical Guidance, (2) Safety of Blood and Blood Products and (3) Public Health.

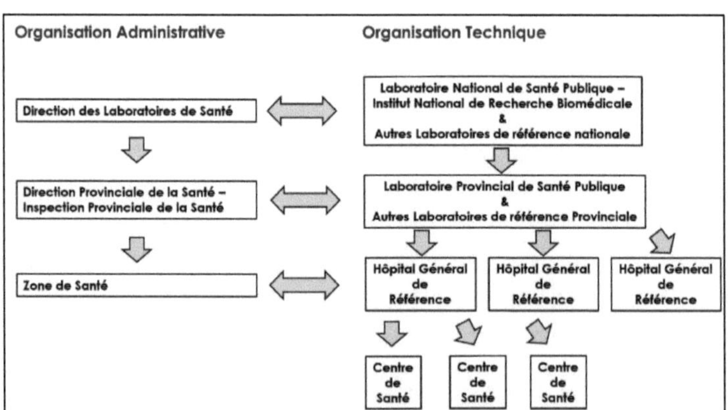

Figure 10: Organisation of the health laboratory sub-sector

Located at the central level of the DRC health system, the DLS relies on the provincial health division (DPS) and the provincial public health laboratory for all specific LBM issues at the intermediate (provincial) level. Within the DPS, it is the office in charge of "Health Information" which, among other things, currently manages the LBM sub-sector with significant support from the provincial public health laboratory (Fig.10).

Several standards documents have been designed and validated by the DLS with the technical and financial support of its many partners and the expertise of its technical arm, the INRB. It should be noted that there is a good working relationship between the DLS and the CNBM, which also contributes its expertise, particularly in the design, drafting and validation of standards documents.

By way of illustration, here are a few standards documents initiated and/or already published by the DLS:

- ✓ Revised health laboratory sub-sector policy (2005)
- ✓ National development plan for the laboratory sub-sector (2012-2016)
- ✓ Training module for service providers on biosafety/biosecurity in the laboratory (2022)
- ✓ Training module for service providers on sample storage and transport in the field of medical biology (2022)
- ✓ National strategic plan for the development of laboratory services (PSNDSL 2021-2025)
- ✓ Laboratory design and functionality guide (2021)
- ✓ Biosafety guidelines (2021)
- ✓ Guidelines for the technical specifications of equipment, materials and consumables and laboratory technical facilities (2021)
- ✓ Biomedical sample collection manual (2022)
- ✓ Training module for service providers on taking biomedical samples (2022)
- ✓ Guide de bonne exécution des analyses (GBEA) (2023)
- ✓ Draft revision of the Decree on the organisation and operation of laboratories in the DRC

- ✓ Draft order approving medical biology analysis reagent distribution companies
- ✓ Draft order laying down the conditions for importing medical devices for in vitro diagnostic use
- ✓ Draft order on the registration and marketing authorisation of in vitro diagnostic medical devices
- ✓ Draft decree on the organisation and operation of establishments importing, distributing and selling in vitro diagnostic medical devices
- ✓ Draft decree on the status of the Lubumbashi provincial public health laboratory
- ✓ Draft revision of the organisation manual for the public health laboratory system
- ✓ Draft interministerial decree on the organisation of the laboratory network in the Democratic Republic of Congo
- ✓ Blood transfusion standards project
- ✓ Draft standardised procedure for blood bank supervision
- ✓ National laboratory quality policy project

2.5.2 *National Institute for Biomedical Research (INRB)*

The Institut National de Recherche Biomédicale (INRB), founded in 1984, is a 70,000 m² facility located at 5345 Avenue de la Démocratie (formerly Huileries) in the commune of Gombe in Kinshasa. As the DRC's national public health laboratory (LNSP), INRB has been a WHO collaborating centre since 2018.

The origins of the INRB date back to the time of President Mobutu, who wanted his country to have a major biomedical centre modelled on the Institut Louis Pasteur in Paris. A national commission, set up in 1975 by Professor NGWETE and chaired by Professor MUYEMBE, was put in charge of the project to create a biomedical research centre modelled on the Institut Louis PASTEUR in Paris.

The old hygiene buildings were refurbished and other additional buildings such as shops, sampling rooms and a virology/animal house were built.

The INRB was created with funding from Franco-Congolese cooperation. It was inaugurated on 8 December 1984 by French President François MITTERRAND and Zaire's first State Commissioner Léon KENGO WA DONDO.

In its early days, INRB was co-managed by French and Zairian biomedical experts. But after the hasty departure of the French aid workers in 1991, due to the unfortunate events of looting, the late Dr KANKIENZA was the first Congolese director to manage the INRB (1991-1998). From 1998 to the present day, Professor Jean-Jacques MUYEMBE TAMFUM has been Director and then "Director General" of the INRB (Fig.11).

During its management, the INRB has undergone significant human and material development. It currently operates in accordance with Prime Ministerial Decree No 13/006 of 22 January 2013, which states that its mission is to contribute to improving the health of the Congolese population by implementing and promoting, throughout the DRC, the biomedical investigations necessary for the research, diagnosis, monitoring, prevention and treatment of human diseases of an epidemic or endemic nature in the DRC (Journal Officiel-54ème year n°3, Présidence RDC 2013).

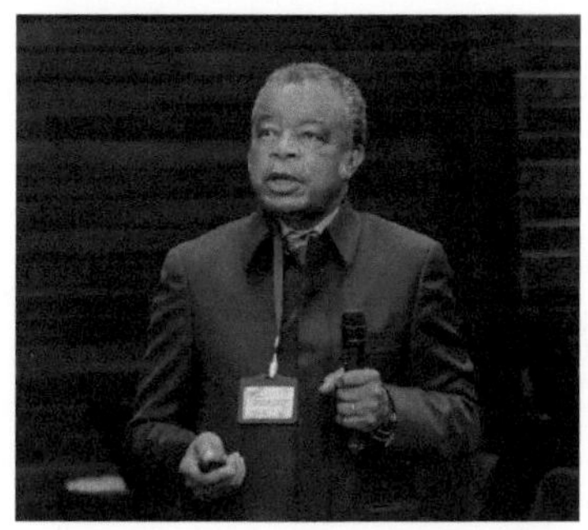

Figure 11: Dr Muyembe Tamfum Jean-Jacques, Professor Emeritus and Director General of INRB, 1998-.

Its scientific staff currently numbers more than 92, including 21 PhDs and some 34 BMs and 29 TLs. The infrastructure comprises several laboratories, including ten BSL-2 laboratories and one BSL-3 laboratory. Its core activities are the performance of biomedical analyses, applied and translational research, the surveillance of communicable diseases and the promotion of professional growth and development. The INRB has continually developed and trained quality researchers and produced outstanding results, most recently concrete efforts in control, prevention and research in the context of the current Ebola epidemic (Fig. 12).

INRB has six main laboratories dedicated to Virology, Parasitology, Bacteriology, Medical Entomology, Clinical Biology and Pathology, including a pathogen genomics laboratory, a bio-bank, a data centre and an animal research centre. Each laboratory has a director and a dedicated staff, including both students and international collaborators. Each laboratory has the basic equipment and space required for optimal research. It is available to faculty, students, post-docs and staff from around the INRB. Due to the structure of INRB, if sharing and access to individual laboratory equipment is required, access is granted upon request and approval of the directors of these laboratories. The INRB's common area includes some major equipment. All staff and researchers have access, on request, to several -80 freezers, liquid nitrogen tanks, centrifuges, water baths, tissue homogenisers, vortexes, incubators, shakers; and all laboratories have access to cold chain equipment such as dry shippers and portable freezers[15]
.

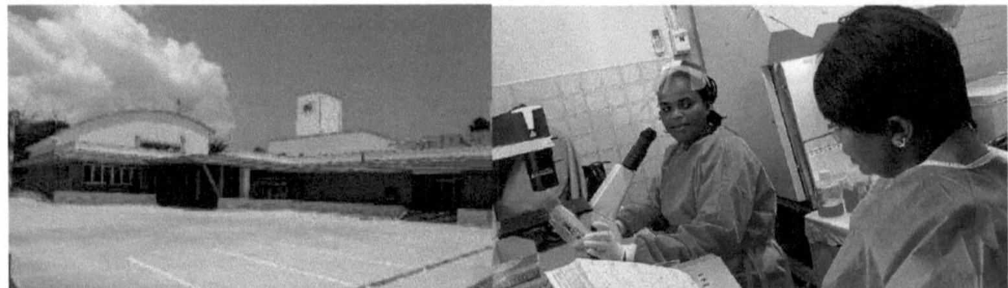

Figure 12: Left: New INRB building housing the BSI-2 and BSL-3 laboratories. On the right, two BM working in the virology laboratory (cell culture bench).

As an LNSP, the INRB plays a leading role in the confirmation and management of epidemics, including Ebola in

[15] Source: 2020 Annual Report of the National Institute for Biomedical Research, Kinshasa

North Kivu, Ituri and Equateur (2015-2022) and COVID-19 (2020-2022).

In addition to government support, the INRB operates and continues to develop thanks to the collaboration and funding of its many partners, represented in Figure 13 by their logos.

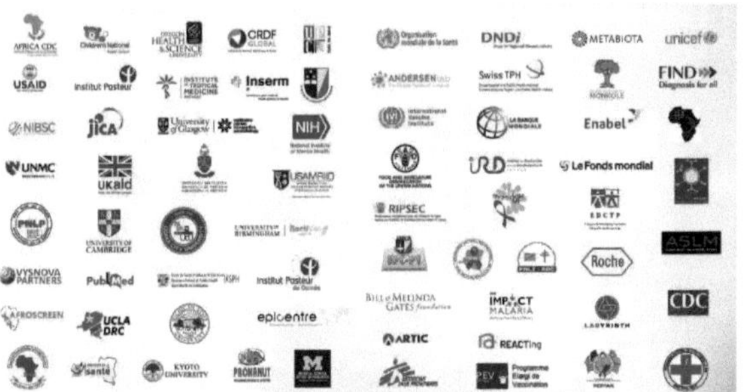

Figure 13: Logos of **INRB** partners

2.5.3 *Cercle de Réflexion en Techniques de Laboratoires (think tank on laboratory techniques)*

The Cercle de Réflexion en Techniques de Laboratoires (CRTL) is a not-for-profit association (ASBL) incorporated under Congolese law, whose main mission is the continuing education and retraining of laboratory professionals in the DRC.

It was set up in 2004 when a group of students on their second laboratory degree course at ISTM-KINSHASA decided to establish a framework for sharing and improving their knowledge of medical biology.

The first name was "cercle de jeune en techniques de laboratoire", but in 2008, at the "Premières Rencontres Nationales de Biologie Technique", the CRTL was adopted as the definitive name.

The LTRC has national coordination, provincial coordination and a number of focal points, including at international level.

Today, under the leadership of its co-ordinator, BM Christian LOBINGA, the CRTL has become an international network of renowned scientific personalities and institutions, and has to its credit numerous activities relating to continuing education, congresses/conferences and other entertainment activities (Fig.

14). These include the "rencontres nationales de biologie Technique" (national meetings on technical biology), continuing education for laboratory professionals in the DRC, support for practical work by medical biology students in a number of ISTMs across the country, and lobbying for equipment for the modern laboratory at ISTM-Kinshasa.

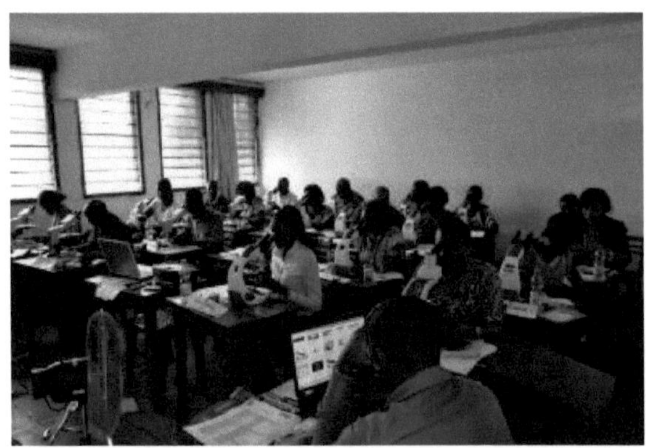

Figure 14a: Training local experts in biological diagnosis, Kinshasa, February 2015 (Source: CRTL)

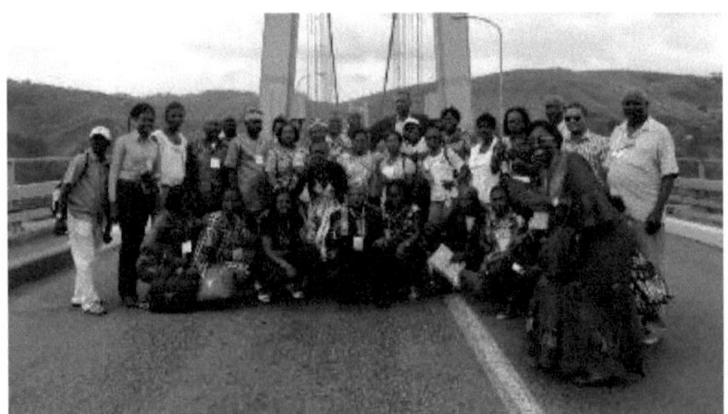

Figure 14b: Participants at the 6th national medical biology meeting, Matadi, October 2015 (Source: CRTL)

The LTRC is currently setting up a continuing education laboratory in Kinshasa.

The LTRC, the CNBM and other institutions involved in medical biology, in particular the DLS, the INRB and the ISTMs, work closely together.

2.5.4 *Dynamics of women medical biologists and laboratory technicians*

The Dynamique des Femmes BM et TL (DFBM) is an organisation that brings together all BM and TL women in the DRC. It was set up in accordance with articles 6 and 24 of the CNBM's statutes. It is a network of women within the CNBM whose aim is to combat the injustices, barriers and inequalities observed in the community in general and in the profession in particular. It also provides a forum for consultation, discussion, sharing, reflection and exchange on the profession.

The idea of creating the DFBM came up at the CNBM's general meeting on 10 March 2013, following a proposal by President Jean-François FEFE. One month later, on 05 April 2013, the DFBM was created during the first conference of women BMs in Africa, at the end of which the DFBM/DRC was appointed president. From its inception until 2020, the DFBM was chaired by WB Sylvie MUSAMBA, and from 2020, she was succeeded by WB Claire BABEKI.

The DFBM coordination committee is made up of Claire BABEKI (President), Véronique NGOMBO (Treasurer), Philomène MUSAMBA (External Relations), Claudine (Secretary), Marina NDILU (Protocol and Logistics), Nancy MAKINFU (Deputy Secretary), Freddy MALEMBE and Emery LUKAKU (Advisers). To date, the DFBM has offices in Muanda, Matadi, Kimpese, Kisangani, Kikwit, Idiofa and Masimanimba.

Apart from the participation of members in all CNBM and CRTL activities, the main activities specific to the DFBM are scientific conferences, mass screening for diseases such as malaria, bio-excursions and health walks (Fig. 15).

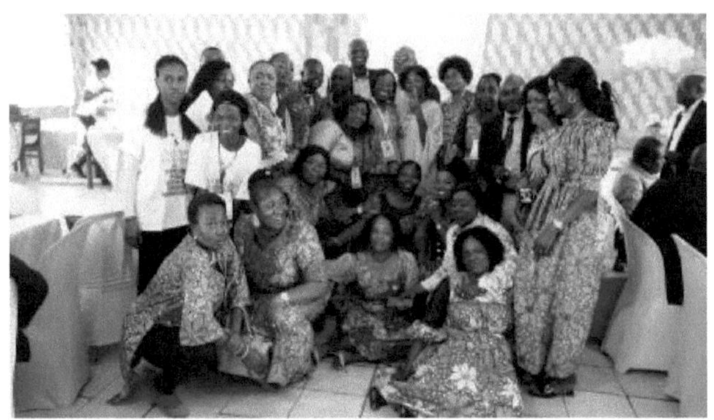

Figure 15: Members of the DFBM during an activity in Kinshasa in 2019 (Source: DFBM)

2.5.5 *Other stakeholders*

- *Association Internationale des Technologistes Biomédicaux (ASSITEB-BIORIF):* has been an NGO since 1972, has official relations with the WHO (1997), the Francophonie (2004) and is a member of RAPF (2011). Its aim is to strengthen laboratory capacity. Its activities focus mainly on training, information, technical assistance, improving working conditions and promoting the value of the professional body. It coordinates a network in 23 countries, particularly in French-speaking Africa and Haiti. The CNBM and ASSITEB-BIORIF have been partners since 2000, and the CNBM has taken part in a number of African meetings sponsored by ASSITEB, notably in Dakar (2004), Brazzaville (2013), Yaoundé (2015) and Bamako (2019).
- *Federation of African Associations of Biomedical Technologists (FASSATEB):* brings together the national associations of TLs and BMs in "French-speaking" Africa. FASSATEB aims to promote biomedical technology. Its specific objectives are (i) to strengthen links between African associations of biomedical technologists; (ii) to improve the quality of technical biology in Africa; (iii) to strengthen the training capacities of African schools of biomedical technologists; (iv) to ensure the continuing education of African biomedical technologists; (v) to perpetuate the Rencontres Africaines de Biologie Technique; (vi) to represent its members in official African and international bodies; and (vii) to participate in biomedical research. The

CNBM has been a member of FASSATEB since its inception in 2009 and currently holds the position of Vice-President, via its national president.

- *Regional Laboratory Professional Association*: brings together all the associations that have signed up to its charter and articles of association. This young association, launched by the African Society of Medical Laboratories (ASLM) in December 2023 in Cape Town/ Republic of South Africa, is in the process of being set up and should have the support of the associations and national councils of all African countries, including the CNBM. The main objectives of this ASLM-CNBM partnership are to :
  - ✓ *To strengthen the development of African laboratory staff* through professional training and capacity-building programmes recognised at both African and national levels in order to meet the needs of human resources in health.
  - ✓ *Strengthening laboratory quality management systems* with a view to international accreditation to transform diagnostic quality and service delivery through the expansion and implementation of the SLIPTA (Stepwise Laboratory Improvement Process Towards Accreditation) programme of the World Health Organization's Regional Office for Africa (WHO-AFRO).
  - ✓ *To promote the LBM profession* on the African continent.
  - ✓ *Establish a South-South cooperation and partnership programme* to provide refresher training opportunities, promote skills transfer and collaboration, and other training opportunities for the young laboratory scientists of the future.
  - ✓ *Organise scientific conferences* as a strategic channel for disseminating the latest LBM information to influence patient care and public health policy, while also encouraging members to attend these conferences.
  - ✓ *Initiate and maintain advocacy* with the government, its partners and donors for the funding of the laboratory system.
- *Medical biologists and laboratory technicians, the brains of medicine:* is a group on "Facebook" made up mainly of BMs and TLs whose aim is to regulate medical practice with scientific

publications and then share news relating to the CNBM for members of the group and the general public.

3 Profile of the laboratory technician and medical biologist (Repository of skills required to practise medical biology)

3.1 *Profile of a laboratory technician*

A TL is responsible for carrying out medical biology examinations and is in charge of all procedures from the pre-analytical stage to the post-analytical stage. The test result delivered by the TL, validated and interpreted by the BM, confirms the diagnosis and allows the clinician to make the important decision in the medical management of the patient. Also, as noted above, the information (result) given by the LBM allows the competent authority to make the important decision within the framework of public health activities.

3.1.1 *Secondary school laboratory technician*

The TL at secondary level (TL A2) receives four years' training at an institution specialising in the health sciences and supervised by the Ministry of Health, Hygiene and Prevention. On completion of their training, TL A2s are competent[16] to: (i) Establish professional communication in the context of biomedical analyses; (ii) Take decisions in the context of biomedical laboratory analyses; (iii) carry out biomedical analyses in parasitology, haematology, bacteriology, biochemistry and immunology (immunohaematology and immunoserology) for diagnosis, screening, therapeutic monitoring and/or health promotion, in accordance with standards, good practice and biosafety rules; (iv) exercise leadership in the management of resources and (v) engage in personal and professional development.

3.1.2 *University-level laboratory technician*

Formerly known as TL A1, university-level TLs are qualified to carry out examinations in the fields of Parasitology, Haematology, Bacteriology, Biochemistry, Immunology, Histopathology, Mycology and Virology. In the hospital environment, they are sometimes required to provide therapeutic

[16] Direction de l'enseignement des sciences de santé/Ministry of Health. Repository of Competences for the Medical Laboratory Technician at secondary level

follow-up in relation to patients and the care team, and may be involved in highly specialised examinations.

In addition, according to the new "LMD system" programme introduced in the DRC, the Ministry of Higher Education and Universities (MINESU) has targeted the following skills[17] :

- Develop simple, clear communication with patients, their families and other healthcare professionals as part of the biologist-patient and biologist-clinician dialogue;
- To study the fundamental concepts of the basic sciences in order to understand the theoretical and practical lessons specific to medical biology;
- Organising the elements needed to carry out biological tests, analysing and processing the results obtained for diagnosis, therapeutic follow-up and prevention;
- To support a policy of quality assurance for biological analyses and management of the biological, chemical, physical and radiological risks associated with its working environment;
- To develop an applied (clinical) or fundamental research activity in the various fields of medical biology in order to help solve a public health problem in the community;
- Managing equipment, materials, consumables, reagents and stocks of products and biological samples in a biomedical analysis laboratory to ensure proper organisation and operation, using IT tools;
- Set up public health intervention mechanisms based on health data obtained from the biomedical analysis laboratory;
- Supporting trainees (trainees in training and laboratory technicians on the job) to build capacity.

It is also capable of using similar analytical methods to carry out examinations in the pharmaceutical industry, veterinary laboratories and other food laboratories.

They must also be familiar with all the concepts and principles of quality management in the LBM, including the management of chemical and biological risks associated with the nature of the

[17] https://www.orientation-pour-tous.fr/metier/technicien-de-laboratoire-medical,14106.html

techniques and products used. They must also be familiar with the regulations applied in these fields, in particular ISO 15189, ISO 15190, etc.

In the DRC, a level A2 TL is qualified and graduated after four years' basic training in medical techniques; this state diploma is issued by the Ministry of Public Health, Hygiene and Prevention. An A1-level TL is qualified after three years' basic university-level training, in accordance with the programme applied by the "Laboratory Techniques" section of the ISTM-Kinshasa and awarded by the MINESU.

This latter course is in the process of being replaced by a Bachelor's degree in Health Sciences, leading to a *"Licence en Techniques de Laboratoire (LTLA)"*, in medical biology, in the field of health sciences. This programme has been officially implemented throughout the DRC by MINESU since the start of the 2021-2022 academic year.

Based on this profile, a TL can also pursue a career as a consultant in public administration, biomedical maintenance technician, in the agri-food, pharmaceutical and cosmetics industry, research assistant, public health specialist, quality and risk management specialist.

However, before starting their career, TLs must register with the National Council of Medical Biologists and Laboratory Technicians of the DRC (CNBM).

3.2 ***Medical biologist profile***

As well as fully meeting the profile of a TL, the BM controls the performance of all medical biology procedures, validates and interprets the results, draws up the report and sends it to the prescriber (clinician, public health authority, etc.) in order to participate in medical diagnosis, patient follow-up and public health activities.

The GP plays a major role in the prevention, diagnosis and treatment of disease. In addition to the dialogue they are expected to maintain with clinicians and public health authorities, they are also appointed advisers to patients, particularly those suffering from pathologies requiring long periods of follow-up and frequent examinations and treatment. To carry out these various functions, the BM must be constantly informed and trained in the latest advances in the biomedical sciences[18] .

The skills and qualities required of a BM include knowledge of the nomenclature of medical biology procedures, mastery of the LBM's analytical techniques and methods, including those relating to the sampling of biological products, scientific and medical knowledge, the ability to validate results, interpret and adapt to rapid changes in techniques and legislation, the ability to implement quality management, including risk management, and team spirit.

In the DRC, the diploma required to become a BM was obtained after five years of basic university training in accordance with the programme applied by the "Laboratory Techniques" section of the ISTM-Kinshasa.

This training programme is currently being replaced by a "*Maîtrise*" *(Master's degree in English)* initiated by MINESU from the start of the 2021-2022 academic year.

The first programme validated by MINESU, the Masters in Clinical Biochemistry and Chemistry (MBCC) is a 2ème cycle course in the Health Sciences, Medical Biology stream. It leads to a Master's degree in "Health Sciences", majoring in "Clinical Biochemistry-Chemistry".

The specific skills covered by this MBCC are :

- Establishing scientific and professional communication in the context of fundamental or applied research;
- Setting up molecular diagnostic methods in the clinical biochemistry-chemistry laboratory;
- Evaluate the mechanisms by which cancers and metabolic diseases occur in the community;
- Assessing the activity of medicinal plants and innovative therapies on metabolic disorders;

---

[18] Medical biologist job: missions, training and salary https://www.studyrama.com/formations/fiches-metiers/sante/biologiste-medical-37484

- Implement the recommendations of the Bioethics Committee on the use of human products and human beings in biomedical research;
- Developing the autonomy of applied (clinical) or fundamental research in the various fields of medical biology.

BMs work in medical and pharmaceutical laboratories, research or teaching organisations, cancer centres, blood transfusion establishments, in the agri-food/pharmaceutical and cosmetics industries, or as advisers in the public administration.

Like the TL, the BM is obliged to register with the CNBM.

The professional development of a BM can lead him or her to become Director of a medical facility, Head of a Provincial Health Division, Public Health Inspector and even University Professor after effective doctoral research leading to a degree at a university.

4 Basic training for laboratory technicians and medical biologists in the Democratic Republic of Congo

There are two successive types of basic training for TLs and BMs in the DRC. The first type of basic training, the post-colonial system, runs respectively from the academic years 1973-1974 to 2020-2021 and 1998-1999 to 2020-2021 for TLs and BMs. The relevant skills and profiles are presented in Chapter 3 and point 4.1 below.

The second type of basic training, in accordance with the LMD system, will start in the 2021-2022 academic year. It includes a Bachelor's degree in Laboratory Techniques and a Master's degree in one of the fields of medical biology, the first being Clinical Biochemistry-Chemistry.

4.1 *Traditional system*

The TL, a graduate in Laboratory Techniques, was trained for three (3) years at university level. This training was reserved for all candidates holding their state diploma, i.e. their baccalaureate. This training included lectures and practical courses, which accounted for forty-six (46) and fifty-four (54) per cent respectively[19] ; the practical work and compulsory work placements during the summer holidays ensured that the TL's skills were particularly "technical".

As for the BM or licencié in Laboratory Techniques, option "*Medical Biology*", the training was also oriented towards technical competence, and was reserved exclusively for graduates in Laboratory Techniques. It included fifty-six (56) percent[20] of practical work, plus approximately five (5) months of work experience during the two (2) years of training.

The skills targeted for the TL and BM included:

[19] ISTM-Kinshasa. Content of the training for the Graduate in Laboratory Techniques. http://istmkin.education/fr/techniques-de-laboratoire/

[20] ISTM-Kinshasa. Contents of the Bachelor of Laboratory Techniques course. http://istmkin.education/fr/techniques-de-laboratoire/

4.1.1 *Laboratory technician*

At the end of their training, graduates in Laboratory Techniques should be able to carry out the following main tasks:

- Collecting biological samples in clinics and in the field for biomedical analyses;
- Technically validate and interpret the results of biomedical analyses;
- Prepare and test reagents, standards and culture media;
- Manage and use the equipment and accessories provided;
- Drawing up statements of requirements and maintaining stock inventories;
- Supervising and managing the staff provided, including trainees.

The TL was also able to work in research, in the pharmaceutical and agri-food industries, in teaching and in public administration relating to public health.

4.1.2 *Medical biologist*

The graduate in Laboratory Techniques, Medical Biology option, should be able to manage a medical laboratory and carry out the following tasks in particular:

- Efficiently monitor the performance of biomedical analyses;
- Biological validation and interpretation of analysis results;
- Coordinate activities in the department and supervise TLs from both a scientific and professional point of view;
- Manage human, financial and material resources effectively;
- Supervising trainees;
- Supervise quality control of analyses, products and reagents;
- Dialogue with stakeholders (patients, clinicians, etc.)

The WB is also capable of playing an important role in epidemiological surveillance, in the pharmaceutical and agri-food industries, in teaching and in public administration relating to public health, higher and university education and scientific research.

4.2 ***Licence- Maîtrise- Doctorat" system ("Medical Biology", a course in the "Health Sciences" field)***

In line with the DRC government's vision of revitalising, requalifying and innovating higher and university education, a number of initiatives have been undertaken in recent years to this end. These include the ESU General Assembly held in Lubumbashi from 6 to 14 September 2021, one of whose recommendations was the development of the LMD reform from the start of the 2021-2022 academic year. Thus, curricular reform to promote the anchoring in coherence with the contextualised normative framework of the LMD system was obvious.

Experts (professors and specialists) from all fields have worked efficiently to produce training offers, including one for the Bachelor's degree in Laboratory Techniques and the other for the Master's degree in Medical Biology, with the *Biochemistry-Clinical Chemistry*, *Haematology-Immuno* Haematology and *Medical Microbiology* courses first on the list[21] .

The competencies relating to these two courses are set out in Chapter 3.

[21] MINESU. Bachelor's and Master's degree models, health sciences field. MINESU-RDC 2021

5 Status and role of laboratory technicians and medical biologists in the Democratic Republic of Congo

There are very few regulations governing the medical biology profession in the DRC. The immediate consequence is the current LBM context characterised by widespread neglect of the LBM sector. Although a significant improvement in the LBM system has been initiated at the central and intermediate levels of the DRC health system, notably with the leadership of the INRB and the Direction des Laboratoires de Santé (DLS), the LBM system in the DRC remains under-performing according to the reports of the few evaluations carried out throughout the country.

One of the few existing documents governing the profession dates from 2003. The practice of medical biology is reserved exclusively for the holder of a qualification or diploma corresponding to six years of secondary school studies for the A2 level TL, three years of studies in the graduate cycle for the A1 level TL, a degree in medical biology for the BM and a basic diploma in Medicine or Pharmacy supplemented by a specialisation in one of the branches of medical biology for doctors and pharmacists respectively[22] .

With the implementation of the LMD system in the ESU, including for the "Health Sciences" field, as well as the numerous developments of the LBM system in the DRC and of LBM-related technology, it is necessary and even urgent to initiate new texts for the practice of medical biology in the DRC. These include

- To update Ministerial Order n°1250/ CAB/MIN/S/CJ/13/2003 of 03/05/2003 on the organisation and operation of health laboratories in the DRC;
- Update the national policy text for the LBM System in the DRC;
- Drawing up the text relating to the status of the DRC's TL and BM.

As for the role, Ministry of Health Order n°1250/ CAB/MIN/S/CJ/13/2003 of 03 May 2003 and other Congolese instructions stipulate that the TL and/or BM is responsible for all

[22] Ministerial decree n°1250/ CAB/MIN/S/CJ/13/2003 of 03/05/2003 on the organisation and operation of health laboratories in the DRC.

activities relating to the analytical process and ensures that they are carried out correctly and meet the fundamental requirements of quality and competence. This mainly involves preparing the patient for the samples; taking the samples, excluding those for which specific training is required; receiving and preparing the samples, including packaging and dispatch where necessary; analysing the samples in accordance with the relevant procedures and instructions, including technical validation of the results; ensuring biological validation of the results by the BM, followed by appropriate information management.

They are also expected to communicate, develop and maintain dialogue with all stakeholders, including (i) other healthcare professionals in medical facilities (pharmaceutical and radiology technicians, physiotherapists, nurses, pharmacists, doctors, surface and administrative technicians, suppliers of IVD products, etc.), (ii) those involved in the epidemiological surveillance of diseases (epidemiologists, anthropologists, nurses, doctors, other public health experts, etc.), (iii) researchers and other players involved in the development of IVD.), (ii) actors involved in the epidemiological surveillance of diseases (epidemiologists, anthropologists, nurses, doctors, other public health experts, etc.), (iii) researchers and other actors involved in the operation of a teaching laboratory in university settings.

6 Workplaces in the profession of laboratory technician and medical biologist.

TL and BM are currently useful in many areas of working life, from health to operational or empirical scientific research. Here are some of the professional environments in which TLs and BMs are used:

6.1 *Medical structure*

In a medical facility (health centre, hospital, clinic, diagnostic centre, public health laboratory), the TLs and BMs are responsible for ensuring that the analytical process is carried out correctly and results are reliable and consistent with the patient's clinical condition.

6.2 *Technical, higher education and university institutions*

With their knowledge and technical skills, TLs and BMs can be in charge of practical and professional work for learners, as well as analyses relating to research undertaken in these environments. The BM can also prepare reagents and culture media or initiate research under the supervision of a certified researcher such as a professor.

The BM, in particular, can undertake and effectively fulfil the role of teacher and/or educational supervisor of students or learners within universities and other higher education institutions in the health sciences, particularly in medical biology.

It should be noted that TLs and BMs are able to complete their training up to the point of defending a doctoral thesis, enabling them to embark on a career as a university professor.

6.3 *Industries*

In the agri-food, pharmaceutical and cosmetics industries, TLs and BMs are responsible for activities relating to the taking and processing of samples, including packaging and dispatch, preparation of equipment, analyses (of food and chemical products), validation and interpretation of results and management of laboratory data.

6.4 ***Public administration***

TLs and BMs provide their expertise in public administration, particularly within ministries and provincial divisions relating to health and scientific research. They are mainly "Advisers", but may also hold positions as "Head of Office", "Head of Division", "Director", "Director General", "Secretary General". Furthermore, TL/BMs are not excluded or prohibited from being active in political life as "Municipal Councillor", "Provincial/National Deputy", "Senator", "Member of the Provincial/National Government" or "President of the Republic".

6.5 ***Governmental and non-governmental organisations***

Project implementation, consultancy and field surveys are increasingly the functions performed by TLs and BMs in national and international governmental and non-governmental organisations. Examples include organisations such as the WHO, the United States Agency for International Development (USAID), the Belgian Development Agency (ENABEL), the Japan International Cooperation Agency (JAICA), the Global Alliance for Vaccines and Immunisation (GAVI), the Clinton Health Access Initiative (CHAI), the International Center for AIDS Care and Treatment (ICAP) and Actions Communautaires SIDA/ Avenir Meilleur pour les Orphelins (ACS/AMO-Congo).

7 Organisation and operation of a medical biology laboratory (Quality and competence requirements)

As elsewhere in the world, in addition to national and regional standards, the DRC's LBM is governed mainly by the international standard ISO 15189, the December 2022 version of which describes the updated requirements concerning quality and competence. It should be noted, however, that very few BMLs in the DRC have implemented the QMS in their organisation and operation.

Overall, the organisation and operation of a laboratory requires infrastructure, equipment and methods,

An MBL should meet, but not be limited to, the following requirements:

7.1 *General requirements*

Broadly speaking, these include impartiality, confidentiality (information management, communication of information, staff responsibilities) and requirements relating to patients.

7.2 *Structural and governance requirements*

An LBM should be recognised as a legal entity headed by a laboratory director with skills, responsibilities and the ability to delegate tasks and/or responsibilities to his or her colleagues.

The activities of an LBM should be clearly described and comply with the requirements based on consultancy services. A structure, via an organisation chart with the definition of authority at each level of responsibility, including quality management. Finally, objectives and policies should be defined, explained to all staff and implemented on an ongoing basis. Risk management should also be in place in accordance with local and/or international standards (ISO 15190: 2020).

7.3 *Resource requirements*

The LBM must have qualified, competent and, to a lesser extent, high-performing staff in order to provide valid day-to-day services. Ongoing training, regular assessment and professional development of staff should be documented and implemented.

The laboratory must operate in appropriate facilities that meet all biological safety and security requirements. Facilities for receiving customers (patients), taking biological samples, analysis, storage and other premises dedicated to administrative and sanitary activities should meet the specific requirements of an MBL, in particular the permanent control of environmental conditions of temperature, humidity and, if necessary, pressure for analysis rooms.

Appropriate equipment, as up to date and efficient as possible, purchased from legally recognised suppliers, selected and assessed regularly, should be used in accordance with verified/validated methods, including local conditions. The aim is to ensure correct operation and prevent contamination or deterioration. In addition, all equipment, where possible, should be calibrated whenever necessary and metrological traceability ensured and documented.

Reagents include all substances purchased commercially or prepared locally (by the LBM itself), standards and controls, culture media, consumables (single-use glassware, pipette tips and other supplies required for medical biology analyses. Like the equipment, the reagents used must be subject to a rigorous procedure for supply, verification/validation, storage, acceptance testing and stock management.

Finally, all the support services needed to manage and carry out its activities must be available and effectively maintained. These include, for example, contracts with the laboratory's users on the one hand and with the operators of the additional requirements relating to off-site medical biology analyses on the other.

Of the products and services provided by external service providers, the LBM must ensure that they are appropriate. For example, the LBM must make its requirements known to subcontracting laboratories and consultants, particularly with regard to the competence of technical staff, analytical procedures and the management of critical results. Finally, the LBM should have procedures for the review and approval of products and services provided by external service providers.

7.4 ***Process requirements***

It is recommended that the LBM reduce, as far as possible, the risks relating to patient management throughout the analytical process. To this end, the use of locally written and validated procedures for each of the related activities is mandatory.

Throughout the pre-analytical process, customers must have access to all relevant information relating to the technical facilities available, instructions on sample collection and handling, patient consent if required, and sample transport and reception.

For the analytical process, the LBM is required to use validated methods that are as universal as possible. To achieve this, the performance specifications for each analytical method must be appropriate to the analysis concerned and its impact on patient care. All documentation, including related procedures, must be accessible to staff. Staff are obliged to comply with instructions and procedures. Finally, skilled and authorised personnel must regularly evaluate the analytical methods used in the LBM's technical platform to ensure that they are still appropriate for the analysis requests received.

Conclusion

Accurate and effective biomedical investigations are essential for preventing, diagnosing and managing disease. The results of analyses produced by the LBM represent the main and indispensable information in a preventive, diagnostic, prognostic and therapeutic approach, including in the implementation of universal health coverage, which requires a fundamental change in the delivery and integration of services in order to meet the diverse needs of communities.

The history of the DRC's TLs and BMs is closely linked to that of the ISTM-Kinshasa and to a number of personalities, including former experts from the WHO, Belgian cooperation and, above all, the pioneering TLs and BMs of the professional association ATELAMEZ, now known as the CNBM.

Many TLs and BMs have developed professionally and are now university professors, experts in national and international governmental and non-governmental organisations, company directors and businessmen/women in the fields of public health and even national politics.

Today, with the implementation of the LMD education system, current and future TL/ BMs have the opportunity, apart from the clinic and public health where they play the most important role, to develop their careers in fields such as university, public administration, industry, business and politics in the DRC.

References

- Linsuke S, Nabazungu G, Ilombe G, Ahuka S et al. Medical laboratories and quality of care: the most neglected area in rural hospitals in the Democratic Republic of Congo. *MAN* 2020
- Horton S, Fleming KA, Kuti M, et al. The top 25 laboratory tests by volume and revenue in five different countries. *Am J Clin Pathol* 2019; 151: 446-51.
- Kenneth A Fleming, Susan Horton, Michael L Wilson, Rifat Atun, et al. The Lancet Commission on diagnostics: transforming access to diagnostics. *Lancet* 2021 Vol 398
- Ministry of Higher and University Education. Maquettes de licence et de maitrise domaine de sciences de la sante. Kinshasa 2021
- International Organization for Standardization. Medical laboratories - Requirements for quality and competence (ISO 15189: 2022). Geneva 2022
- Ministry of Public Health, Hygiene and Prevention. Direction des laboratoires de Santé. Guide de bonne exécution des analyses de biologie médicale. Kinshasa, DRC 2012.
- Tawite S, Mukadi P. Preliminary report of the assessment of the specimen reference system in Equateur Province, Democratic Republic of Congo. International center for AIDS care and treatment program 2022 (Unpublished)
- Ministry of Public Health, Hygiene and Prevention. Arrêté Ministériel N°CAB/FP/JMK/PP/044/2003 du 28 mars 2003 portant création du laboratoire médical. Kinshasa 2003
- Ministry of Public Health, Hygiene and Prevention. Arrêté n°1250/ CAB/MIN/S/CJ/13/2003 du 03/05/2003 portant organisation et fonctionnement des laboratoires de santé en République Démocratique du Congo. Kinshasa 2003
- Lufuluabo J, Planification, organisation et administration d'un service national de laboratoire de santé publique. Echos des Tropiques, ISBN: 99951-51-25-1, Kinshasa, 2021
- National Institute for Biomedical Research. Annual report. Kinshasa 2020

- World Health Organization (WHO). Manual of basic laboratory techniques. WHO, Geneva 1982
- World Health Organisation (WHO). Laboratory Quality Management System, Training Tool. WHO, Geneva 2012
- Butel MJ, Cals MJ. Repository of skills required to practise medical biology. 2008
- Canadian Institute for Health Information. Medical Laboratory Technologists and Their Workplace. Québec, 2010
- Democratic Republic of Congo, Official Journal. Constitution of the Democratic Republic of Congo, Amended by Law No. 11/002 of 20 January 2011 revising certain articles of the Constitution of the Democratic Republic of Congo of 18 February 2006. Kinshasa 2011
- Institut Supérieur de Techniques Médicales. Contenu de la formation du Gradué en Techniques de Laboratoire. ISTM-Kinshasa http://istmkin.education/fr/techniques-de-laboratoire/ (Page consulted on 19 January 2023)
- Institut Supérieur de Techniques Médicales. Contents of the training for the Bachelor's degree in Laboratory Techniques. http://istmkin.education/fr/techniques-de-laboratoire/ (Page consulted on 19 January 2023)
- Ministry of Public Health, Hygiene and Prevention. Law No. 18/035 of 13 December 2018 establishing the fundamental principles relating to the organisation of Public Health in the Democratic Republic of Congo. Kinshasa 2018
- Presidency of the Republic, Decree No. 13/006 of 22 January 2013 on the creation, organisation and operation of a public establishment called the "Institut National de Recherche Biomédicale", abbreviated to "I.N.R.B". Kinshasa 2013
- National Council of Medical Biologists and Laboratory Technicians. Statuts. Kinshasa 2019
- Ministry of Public Health, Hygiene and Prevention. National Health Development Plan (PNDS) 2011-2015. Kinshasa 2010
- Ministry of Public Health, Hygiene and Prevention. Organisation du Système des Laboratoires de Santé Publique dans le cadre de la surveillance épidémiologique, March 2005

- Nkengasong JN, Nsubuga P, Nwanyanwu O, et al. Laboratory systems and services are critical in global health, *Am J Clin Path*. 2010;134;368-73.
- https://www.studyrama.com/formations/fiches-metiers/sante/biologiste-medical-37484#formations Pages viewed on 14 April 2023

Other resources

- Presentations at the 43ème CNBM anniversary: 20 March 2021 at INPESS, Kinshasa
- Interviews with the co-founding members of ATELAMEZ, presidents and other members of successive national committees since the first committee was set up on Saturday 18 March 1978 (Alois BATANGILAYI), then Denis KANDOLO KAKONGO, Papy MUWOYA, Pascal MANUELE (2014- 2018) and Blandin BOKABELA (2018-2022).

Appendix

Pioneers of medical biology in the Democratic Republic of Congo interviewed during the writing of this book

Names	Description	Function/ Association
MUSHIYA WA KALONJI Elisabeth (1ère Graduating class/ 1976)	Medical biologist in charge of monitoring priority diseases at INRB	Assistant Secretary/ ATELAMEZ, 1978- 1986
LUFULUABO KASUYI Jean (1ère Graduating class/ 1976)	Professor at ISTM-Kinshasa	Scientific advisor, CNBM, 2008- to date
KANDOLO KAKONGO Dénis (1ère Graduation/ 1976)	Professor at ISTM-Kinshasa and Rector of Kalima University	President/ ATELAMEZ-CNTL, CNBM, 1986- 2001
BATANGILAYI MESU Aloïs (1ère Graduating class/ 1976)	Quality Manager at the National Blood Transfusion Centre, Kinshasa	Chairman/ ATELAMEZ, 1978- 1986
KABENGELE WA KABENGE Marcel (1ère Graduation/ 1976)	Head of Research at the ISTM-Kinshasa and researcher at the Centre Régional d'Etudes Nucléaires de Kinshasa (Kinshasa Regional Centre for Nuclear Studies)	Honorary Secretary ATELAMEZ, 1978- 1986
BOKABELA Blandin (12ème Graduating class/ 1988)	Blood Bank Manager, Cliniques Universitaires de Kinshasa LBM technical auditor	President CNBM, 2018-
MUWOYA Ndjungayane Papy (9ème graduating class/ 1985)	Head of Laboratory MONUSCO	President CNTL- CNBM, 2001 - 2014
Fefe BALEKA (9ème graduating class/ 1985)	Medico-technical coordinator/ Clinique Ngaliema Training Officer/ National Tuberculosis Control Programme Medico-Technical Director/ CHIP	Provincial President CNBM- Kinshasa, 1991-2016

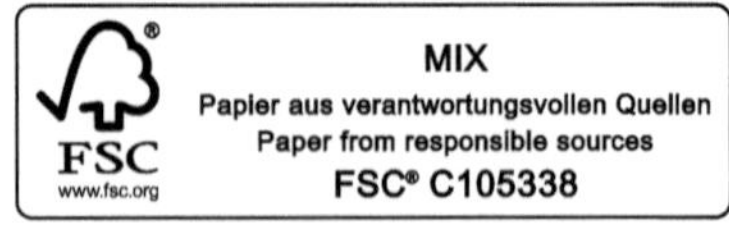

Printed by Books on Demand GmbH, Norderstedt / Germany